FEB 2024

BREAK
THE
CYCLE

BREAK
THE
CYCLE

A Guide to Healing
Intergenerational Trauma

DR. MARIEL BUQUÉ

DUTTON

DUTTON

An imprint of Penguin Random House LLC
penguinrandomhouse.com

Copyright © 2024 by Mariel Buqué
Penguin Random House supports copyright. Copyright fuels creativity, encourages diverse voices, promotes free speech, and creates a vibrant culture. Thank you for buying an authorized edition of this book and for complying with copyright laws by not reproducing, scanning, or distributing any part of it in any form without permission. You are supporting writers and allowing Penguin Random House to continue to publish books for every reader.

DUTTON and the D colophon are registered trademarks of Penguin Random House LLC.

LIBRARY OF CONGRESS CATALOGING-IN-PUBLICATION DATA

Names: Buqué, Mariel, author.
Title: Break the cycle: a guide to healing intergenerational trauma / Dr. Mariel Buqué.
Description: New York : Dutton, [2024] | Includes bibliographical references and index.
Identifiers: LCCN 2023043198 (print) | LCCN 2023043199 (ebook) |
ISBN 9780593472491 (hardcover) | ISBN 9780593472514 (ebook) |
Subjects: LCSH: Families—Mental health. | Psychic trauma—Treatment. | Holistic medicine.
Classification: LCC RC455.4.F3 B87 2024 (print) | LCC RC455.4.F3 (ebook) |
DDC 616.85/21—dc23/eng/20231020
LC record available at https://lccn.loc.gov/2023043198
LC ebook record available at https://lccn.loc.gov/2023043199

Printed in the United States of America
1st Printing

Illustration by Madeline Kloepper

While the author has made every effort to provide accurate telephone numbers, internet addresses, and other contact information at the time of publication, neither the publisher nor the author assumes any responsibility for errors or for changes that occur after publication. Further, the publisher does not have any control over and does not assume any responsibility for author or third-party websites or their content.

All names and identifying characteristics have been changed to protect the privacy of the individuals involved.

For my sister, Lady.
Thank you for modeling for me how to break cycles
with love at the center. May we continue to
live out our intergenerational legacy.
I love you *más*.

Contents

Sensitivity Acknowledgment

In the pages of this book, I have done my very best to offer as much inclusion to diverse experiences as is within my realm of knowledge. I aimed to be as responsive and actionable in my language and approach as I am able. Any text will have limitations, but I hope that you will feel seen and validated through reading this book. If any part of your experience doesn't hold true in what I have reflected here, I hope you can take what you can from this book and attend to the pieces that do offer you healing.

A Note about Professional Emotional Help

Contacting a professional, like a psychotherapist, to help walk you through your emotions is sometimes necessary when working through intergenerational trauma. This is especially so if you feel you could use the help in processing any trauma. If working with a therapist is of interest or accessible to you, it's a good rule of thumb to do any healing work that is centered on trauma with a licensed professional who is trauma trained and trauma responsive.

If you or someone you love is undergoing a cycle of abuse and is looking for help, there are some resources that can be helpful:

- Calling local crisis teams if someone's life is in danger
- The International List of Sexual & Domestic Violence Agencies: hotpeachpages.net

INTRODUCTION

My grandmother, my mother, and I all grew up in poverty. My grand-mother lived almost all her life in the tiny town of Barahona, Domini-can Republic (DR). I remember at the age of ten walking over a mile with her to collect five gallons of water from a small spring because neither her home nor her village had running water, a basic necessity that so many of us take for granted. With her petite four-foot-five-inch frame, my grandmother carried those five gallons all the way back to her tiny home, holding my hand while steadily balancing the heavy bucket on her head, preserving every drop of the water she had collected for her family. It's an image that I can never erase from my mind because it was both jarring and humbling to see just how little she had and yet how resourceful she could be. She would salvage not only every drop of water, but also every bit of food, the very last of the toiletries she could afford, and every last item of clothing. She understood that this level of preservation was necessary for survival. She had to live in survival mode her entire life, but despite it, she held on to so much resilience. Because of my grandmother, I learned about the great value of preserv-ing not only water but every small thing that we owned. Nothing could go to waste. Because of her, I also learned how capable of mental strength and joy I, too, could be.

My mother, who migrated to the United States at the age of forty with her two young daughters, has held on to that spirit of preservation her entire life. My mother has always been a *keeper*. She keeps everything, sometimes for decades, even if it is no longer functional. We lived in a low-income community in Newark, New Jersey, for most of my life, but my mother always saw us as having so much, because her childhood back in Barahona had taught her what it was to have next to nothing. So, whenever we grew out of our clothes, or an appliance broke, or there were household items we were no longer using, they wouldn't get thrown away. Instead, they would be packed away neatly in a box, and years later, when we'd have enough money to send these things to our family, they would be shipped to the DR. Over the years, boxes containing decades of saved items piled up in our home. But gradually, I learned that what was truly being preserved in those boxes wasn't worn clothing or a broken toaster—it was my mother's fear of being left with nothing. This comes from a scarcity mindset, driven by true scarcity in her childhood, which became embedded as a fear of not being able to survive, and the guilt of not being able to help her family do the same.

I now live a comfortable life, as does my mom, but I've often found myself holding on to things that I don't need, the same way she did. I have lived with that same fear and guilt. If I were to throw items away rather than donating them or sending them to the DR, I would be riddled with guilt. If I didn't use something to the last drop, I would find my inner self nudging me, whispering to me that I was being wasteful and that I might need it, just in case someday I'm left with nothing. Even though I have always had running water in my home, I still lived with my grandmother's fear that someday the water would run out. I held on to that same panic. My family's fear had been transferred onto me, and in some strange way, I have felt a deep loyalty to them when I carefully preserved things. In doing so, I felt I was honoring them. It took a long time to realize that my loyalty came at a psychological cost.

Fortunately, because I have been able to break the cycle of what I have come to understand is intergenerational trauma, I have been able to shake off the guilt and fear almost entirely. And I want other people who are suffering to be able to do the same, to shake off their loyalty to pain and transition to a place of emotional freedom. In order to do that, however, those suffering must first recognize and heal through the intergenerational ties that they have to their own family's lineage of pain. It is not easy, but it is possible, and the abundance that can come from this healing is beautiful and worth the effort.

But how did I come to identify this pain as intergenerational trauma? And what *is* intergenerational trauma, exactly?

It all started during my years in the Adult Outpatient Psychiatry Clinic of Columbia University's Irving Medical Center, where I received my doctoral training. I was with a client, and the session . . . well, it was rough. Very few things in this world are as frustrating to a mental health clinician than reaching what feels like a dead end in a session—and that's exactly where my client and I had arrived. It was a moment in which we had to sit with a suffocating sense of helplessness that filled the room. I felt I had nothing else to offer my client, because my training, as robust as it was, hadn't prepared me for what was happening in this moment.

I suddenly understood the reason for the fog. My client was the bearer of intergenerational guilt, sadness, grief, depression, anxiety—the list goes on and on. We weren't just working through my client's pain. We were working on the emotional burdens of my client's family and ancestors, people who weren't in the room with us during session, and perhaps who weren't even alive anymore. This was a *major* therapeutic challenge. No traditional training in Western psychology has adequately prepared any of us mental health clinicians to treat patients for intergenerational trauma. There is no guidebook for when clients come to us with the emotional wounds of an entire lineage of family members.

I felt the weight of the generations that came into that therapy session with my client. At that point in our therapeutic journey, the only way to cut through that thick fog was to face the generations of pain we were dealing with. And as hard as it was, I knew we had to deepen the work.

The realizations that came from this session changed me forever. I thought about generational healing every day from that moment on. I thought about how a person could carry traumas that weren't experienced in their lifetime. I wondered about how trauma could be transmittable from one person to another. I grew curious about the different ways in which intergenerational trauma could be handed down. Did it just look like this client's story, or were there other variations that can show up in our lives? My mind was spinning trying to find answers. I felt the pressure of helping my client feel better but also the pressure as a clinician to find a healing protocol that could help countless other people who were suffering this way. That session was a turning point in how I approached my clinical work. My mission blossomed: I found my purpose to better understand what to do when a person came in with an entire family's emotional pain and a desperation to heal such pain.

Like the scientist that I am, I decided to investigate what practices needed to be put in place to help people—meaning, people like you and me—heal generations of wounding, to shed the trauma responses that our families and communities have been experiencing and replace these trauma responses with healthy and adaptive coping strategies.

Intergenerational trauma is the only category of emotional trauma that transcends generations and could be experienced by multiple members of your family. But how has this trauma moved through the generations of your family to reach you? We now know that there are two modes of transmission. The first is through your *biology*, or more specifically, through your gene expressions, which are inherited from each parent. That means that if either of your parents experienced trauma, that trauma could have altered them so fundamentally as to appear in their genetic code. You may have inherited those genes, making you more vulnerable to stress and trauma.

The second mode of transmission is through experiences that impact your *psychology*, like misattunement with caregivers, invalidation, harmful relationships, extreme adversity, oppression, and suffering that you experience in your own lifetime. This is how trauma is passed from a caregiver to a child or from society to a person, through *behaviors and practices*.

Now, intergenerational trauma can be broken, and that genetic inheritance doesn't need to be passed down further, hence the reason we're here, healing through these pages. But let's consider what happens when a person carries those biological emotional vulnerabilities *and* did not have the healthy and safe emotional foundation that they needed. That's when the cycle of trauma can become evident. That is when we can say you're living with intergenerational trauma. And although this type of trauma may have originated somewhere in your family lineage through an event experienced by one individual, its psychological, behavioral, and emotional repercussions may impact multiple family members and even entire communities across generations.

Intergenerational trauma is a wounding of the soul. It's a multilevel emotional injury that impacts a person's mind (their thoughts and emotions), body (the way they carry suffering physically), and spirit (a disruption in their inner knowing and connection with others). I realized, therefore, that healing must also be multidimensional. It has to heal every layer of a person in mind-body-spirit—meaning, it has to heal their soul.

Because of this, I embrace holistic healing methods. When I say holistic healing methods, I'm referring to a wide range of practices that help heal the whole person. Holistic therapy, which is the type of therapeutic approach I take in healing traumas, aligns all parts of the person. It understands that we are a sum of all our parts and that our healing should seek to integrate us and help us feel whole. When one aspect of our health is off, the others also suffer. When we target the whole person in the healing process, we help heal the whole person.

The field of psychology hasn't yet caught up to embrace holistic methods of healing emotional wounds, but I was fortunate to train in a three-year clinical fellowship that allowed me to work with seasoned psychologists who stepped outside the box. They knew to nurture their clients through less conventional, holistic, ancestral, and integrative mental health modalities. Through that fellowship and in my own work over the years, I have learned that if you let one part of a person carry the wound—attending to the mind but not the body, for example—you risk shifting the pain from one dimension to another, but you will not offer full healing.

I knew when I set out on my mission to learn everything I could about how to identify and treat intergenerational trauma, that healing something so complex would require the traditional trauma methodologies that I had been trained to provide, but also something more nuanced, something with greater depth. That something is the tailored approach that I have developed after years of study and that I have employed with my clients. And my approach works.

With this book, I will, for the first time, collect all my teachings to offer you a definitive guide to healing intergenerational trauma.

This book follows a flow that is similar to how I work with my clients. Within each chapter, I'll provide you with an in-depth orientation to each aspect of intergenerational healing, and then I will offer a practice to help you focus and apply the work. So, as you read, you will see that I offer you concrete knowledge with multiple points of guidance to integrate each lesson into your own life, followed by a set of practices for breaking the cycle at the end of each chapter. These practices are holistic and therapeutic. Within each exercise, I will help you work through that specific chapter's focus. That way, I can help you absorb the content in a more profound way.

For each exercise, you also have the option to work on your own or together with someone else. Healing can be very special when done in community, so if you decide to find a partner or gather a group of fellow cycle breakers to do this work with, each end-of-chapter exercise can be devoted to your work in unison. So, whether you choose to work on your own or with others, you have options on how to approach your healing.

Additionally, each section has its own sound bath meditation. Sound baths are an ancient practice that can help relax your mind and body. To help orient you further, I will cover sound baths in greater depth in chapter 1.

Taken together, these will be tools to add to your toolbox. They are there to guide you. Know that this healing journey is your own, so lean into what works for you.

Now let's give you an overview of what to look forward to in the chapters ahead. I start by laying the foundation of what intergenerational trauma is and how it has found its way into your life. Part 1, "What You Inherited," is made up of five chapters. In each of these chapters, we take a deep dive into what intergenerational trauma really is and how a person inherits emotional pain from their parents, grandparents, ancestors, and community. You will also learn how the mind, body, and spirit are all impacted by this inheritance, and the intergenerational resilience you hold despite it all. In chapter 1, "You Are a Cycle Breaker," we begin with acknowledging your role in breaking cycles. I will offer you a guide for preparing for the hard and necessary work ahead, so you have the tools you need to keep steady as you heal. In chapter 2, "Your Intergenerational Higher Self," we dive into generational wisdom by focusing on your innate cycle-breaking abilities and on your ancestral insight, which act as guides for you to always return to. We will then engage in a practice that can help you connect with your intergenerational higher self. In chapter 3, "Your Body Remembers Your Trauma," I will help you understand how intergenerational trauma is felt in the body and the multiple ways in which chronic illness is connected to generations of stress. We will wrap up by breaking the cycle through a practice that will help decrease your stress response and balance your hormones. Chapter 4, "Unhealed Trauma and You," is where we begin the journey to explore the question "How do you know you are working with intergenerational trauma?" In this chapter, I will provide you with an Intergenerational Trauma Healing Assessment that is designed to help you dig deeper into your lineage's history of trauma. This will function as the first mapping of the intergenerational trauma in your life. We then transition to chapter 5, "A Genetic Inheritance," where I help you understand the role your genes and cells play in the transmission of trauma. I will guide you through an understanding of how your trauma is wired together with your family's trauma, and to that end, I will help you develop your own Intergenerational Trauma Tree, which you can build on your own or with others.

In part 2 of this book, "There Are Layers to This," I cover exactly that: the layers of pain and the layers of healing. In this section, I introduce new, intergenerational ways to look at your nervous system, your inner child, cycles of abuse, and the ways that cultural values keep trauma floating from generation to generation. Chapter 6, "Your Intergenerational Nervous System," is where you'll gain wider knowledge of the role of triggers, memories, and your nervous system. I will then take you through a practice to help you relax your nervous system and alleviate how you respond to stress. In chapter 7, "Your Intergenerational Inner Child," I will help you understand how the unresolved inner child in your parents becomes the inner child in you. It is recycled. I will introduce you to an Intergenerational Adverse Experiences Questionnaire to help you understand how your childhood and your parents' childhoods are intertwined, followed by an intergenerational reparenting exercise. In chapter 8, "Intergenerational Cycles of Abuse," I offer you one of the best armors against continuing cycles of abuse: knowledge. But we won't stop there; I will also equip you with a cycle-breaking tool that you can use to help you through challenging relationship dynamics. And in the final chapter of part 2, chapter 9, "When Collective Trauma Enters Your Home," we discuss collective trauma and the multiple ways in which natural disasters, cultural norms, and institutional practices contribute to keeping trauma alive in your lineage. I will guide you through a practice that will help you reflect on how internalized ideas feed our collective trauma and invite you to extend your healing out to others in your communities.

Part 3, "Alchemizing Your Legacy," is where we really start cementing your cycle-breaker identity. This final part of the book consists of three chapters, which will guide you through grief, the embodiment of intergenerational post-traumatic growth, and the creation of your intergenerational legacy. In chapter 10, "Grieving Your Traumatic Lineage," I will be helping you understand the reasons why family secrets keep going, help you start releasing shame, and provide you with a technique for having difficult conversations about intergenerational trauma with those closest to you. In chapter 11, "Embodying Generational Resilience," I will help you learn how, as a cycle breaker, you can engage in intergenerational post-traumatic growth. Through our Breaking the Cycle practice, you will learn to increase your generational resilience. Our final chapter, chapter 12, "Leaving a Generational Legacy," will help you absorb a cycle breaker approach to life that can positively impact future generations. We will cover how cycle breakers parent their children and ways in which you can adopt a parenting approach that takes into consideration the impact you wish to leave on this world. We will complete this chapter with our last practice, which will help you create alchemy in your legacy process.

This is a comprehensive recipe to shedding intergenerational trauma and an immersive orientation into how to do this work. And it is here for you, to help you step into the intergenerational legacy that lives in you.

I wrote this book for you to learn from it *and* practice from it. It's not just a book you read, but one you apply to your daily life. Since that's the approach, I encourage you to keep a designated notebook and writing materials close by. I will be recommending a number of different exercises, reflection questions, and writing prompts to help you explore and express your feelings as we undertake the work of cycle breaking together. A journal is a key tool for that work.

Throughout this book, you will see me refer to the cycle breaker. That is you. The one who decided to break the cycle. I am grateful that you're here, deciding to heal and stepping into your intergenerational legacy. My wish is that you leave behind the heavy weight that you've been carrying. That you realize that you no longer need to carry this heaviness in order to feel alive; rather, that aliveness can be found in moments of ease and peace. My hope is that you become a cycle breaker of intergenerational trauma and shift your lineage into intergenerational abundance.

Let's start healing.

With love,
Dr. Mariel Buqué

PART I

What You Inherited

CHAPTER I

You Are a Cycle Breaker

It's up to us to break generational curses. When they say, "It runs in the family," you tell them, "This is where it runs out."
—Unknown

If you're reading this book, chances are you are a cycle breaker. You are the person who has decided to create a different legacy for your family and community than the one you inherited, by shifting the ways in which you show up in the world. Your healing quest is not just about you. It has collective motivation. You send ripples of healing backward and forward by becoming a cycle breaker. It's a heavy task and one that, when chosen, or when it chooses you, has the power to liberate your lineage.

Cycle breaking comes with a great reward. It takes some time to get to the reward, but when you do get there, you feel the lightness of inner peace. You deserve to feel that lightness, to feel emotional freedom and no longer carry intergenerational burdens. Cycle breaking is how we put down that baggage of the past and step into a better future. Cycle breakers *choose* to be cycle breakers. It is an active, long-term decision. For you, that choice may have come after seeing the hurt that your family and communities have had to endure and no longer accepting that it must be passed down to the next generation. Or it could stem from your wish to create a different legacy for you and your lineage. One thing is for sure—cycle breakers across the world have one definitive goal in mind: to make sure that repeated generational patterns end with them. By reading this book, you are taking a huge step toward that goal.

Being a cycle breaker is a multitier, multitask, multigenerational quest toward peace. It's peace for you, those who came before you, those who will come after you, your community, and the global culture. Shifting into someone who embodies this mindset is shifting into someone who possesses the inner knowing that this peace is worth fighting for.

Many cycle breakers don't know to identify themselves as such. They just know in their spirit that things must be different. They decide to shift the narrative and welcome opportunity for ease, happiness, and health into their lives. They think of their children's lives and wish a different experience for them than what they had themselves. They think of how much suffering their family has gone through and feel a duty to change that and heal the trauma that plagues their lineage. They see ways in which their communities are unwell and feel motivated to make a change at the community level. They see the global impact of traumatic experiences and want to shift the way things are to create a better global community for us all. They see no other way forward but the way of healing. So they walk through life in active resistance to the status quo. They enter daily battles to fight against what they were taught or how they were treated. To do so, they go off intuition, faith, and courage in order to create a cycle-breaking process that, in hindsight, they're able to see was a powerful course correction for them and everyone around them. Cycle breakers do all these things, which means that you may already be doing these things as well, even if you have never claimed the title of cycle breaker before this moment. You may be at the very beginning of your cycle-breaking journey, and that is just as powerful.

Cycle breakers are not all the same. The combination of these characteristics will vary from person to person, so you may want to grab your journal to write down any that resonate with you. Being a cycle breaker means you:

- See the generational wisdom and resilience that flows through you
- Choose to disrupt trauma responses in your lineage
- Acknowledge your part in keeping cycles going
- Are willing to do the inner work to cut the cord of pain
- Are willing to assume the consequences of disrupting those patterns
- Employ daily mind-based practices to stay conscious of your emotional experiences
- Maintain a lifestyle that influences your body, and particularly your epigenome (the chemical changes in your DNA that can be transmittable intergenerationally), in a positive way
- Ground yourself in spirit-based practices to regenerate your soul
- Acknowledge that your DNA is not your destiny
- Are no longer willing to live in a mindset that upholds the idea that you embody a genetic deficit but, rather, are going to shift to a mindset that embraces genetic abundance
- Are willing to make adjustments to exist in a body that can help you absorb stress better
- See the souls in your community as an extension of your own and treat them accordingly
- Disrupt systemic inequities that promote collective traumas that keep feeding cycles
- Are willing to spread healing knowledge to others so we can all more fully heal in this generation
- See yourself as a living ancestor who has influence over future generations
- Have determined that the cycle of inherited trauma ends with you

One, some, or all of these characteristics may resonate with you as a cycle breaker. Your brand of cycle breaking will be unique to you. Take a moment to reflect on that and ask yourself, "What are my cycle-breaking qualities?" Once you do, keep reading, because throughout this book, you will learn what you, a cycle breaker, have the power to achieve.

My mission is to help you honor the work you already feel compelled to do. To give you tools to help you navigate the heavy emotions and hard conversations you'll want to have with yourself and with your family or community members. I hope to supplement and guide you, and be a voice of understanding for you, as you carry on with the courageous work of cycle breaking that you were born to do.

But How Do You Know You're Ready?

Every cycle breaker is different. However, one thing is the same for us all: no cycle breaker will ever feel fully ready to break the cycle. That's because there is no perfect time, feeling, or clue that will let you know when to act.

One of my clients once had a dream that his ancestor came to him as a blue aura light. My client didn't *hear* his ancestor speak to him during the dream but rather *felt* his ancestor convey, "You must go and fight the battle." His interpretation of this dream is what shifted his readiness. It wasn't anything he planned. It was a subconscious understanding that ancestors were with him and that he was ready for the fight ahead.

The mind and body are vehicles to the soul's higher consciousness, so it's important that we listen carefully to our subconscious. My call to action also came in a dream. It was a message from a living ancestor, my father, who told me, "My child, it is time." This came during a time in my life when I felt like I couldn't mobilize anything. I didn't feel ready.

My impostor syndrome—an intergenerational lie I had absorbed for many decades—was crippling my self-confidence. Impostor syndrome is the feeling that you are a fraud or don't belong in certain spaces, which is driven by the act of being cast out of these spaces for generations. But my interpretation of this dream helped me shift my mindset. I was open to receiving my father's message, which signaled for me the start of the cycle-breaking journey I am on now.

Maybe you have already received a sign or a signal that is preparing you for your own quest to stand in your intergenerational higher self. Maybe it isn't someone else's voice or aura, but your own internal voice speaking to you. If you are here, trust that your soul is ready.

Healing Through Holistic Practices

Remember, one expression of my family's intergenerational trauma was to preserve all possessions because we were in a prolonged survival mode. I realized I was breaking the cycle when I was able to let go of a precious item, my grandmother's mug. It was a beautiful white mug, painted red on the inside, with a little spoon to match and a hole on the handle to hold the spoon. She had sent it to me, with love, in a family member's luggage from the Dominican Republic. Knowing how little my grandmother had, I was so moved and it meant so much to me that she would gather whatever resources she could to reach my home and heart with this gift. I drank from this mug every single day for years. I oftentimes meditated on my grandmother's words and voice while holding my mug with my favorite tea filling it. It was such a central piece in my home. But one day, the mug broke into too many pieces to repair. What hurt even more was that this happened only a few months after my grandmother had passed. The one item I had that created a bridge of connection between us was broken. I was devastated and I felt deep guilt. I felt guilty for not preserving the mug that she had worked so hard to give me. And of course, since fear of loss was also a part of my wounded experience, I was afraid that without this physical item to connect us, I could lose my sacred spiritual connection to her as well, something that was so deeply grounding to me.

I knew intuitively what I needed to do. A part of me even felt that it was my grandmother who helped me know how to heal through this moment. Because trauma manifests in the soul, I had to take steps to heal my whole self if I wanted to move forward.

In my mind, I had to challenge my fear of losing my connection to her and remind myself of all the ways in which I will forever remain tied to her. In my body, I had to take deep breaths, with a focus on my heart, in order to heal the brokenheartedness that was manifesting through bodily aches. For my spirit, I decided to start writing ancestral letters to my grandmother. It elevated my connection to her and continues to do so until this very day.

This experience also informed my approach to my work with clients. Writing letters to ancestors became a tool that I would utilize with my clients who hoped to stay connected to their loved one's ancestral love and wisdom. We did the work of healing the challenging thoughts and feelings that their predecessors couldn't bear to deal with (healing the mind), we worked on shedding the ways their body was remembering these traumas (healing the body), and we worked to help them feel grounded and reconnected (healing the spirit). It was layered, holistic, and deep-rooted work. Breaking the cycle meant healing from the experiences that had become planted in the souls of their families, and now in their own. It was, and continues to be, the only way to sort through the layers of pain that are left behind in the wake of intergenerational trauma. And it's the way I hope we can work together through the pages in this book. Attending to the mind, but leaving the body and spirit still wounded, will leave you in the same place of emotional pain that you and your ancestors have been in for ages. I don't want this for you. I want you to experience the fullness of healing and true emotional liberation. Through the practice of mental holism, which in the medical world means "treating the whole person," we are working to heal the whole you. We will take a holistic healing approach to honor the multiple ways in which you have experienced hurt.

Getting Ready to Do the Work

With intergenerational trauma, there can be so much more than meets the eye. Most people who I have had the deep honor to work with throughout the years have had layers of trauma that needed to be peeled back. They oftentimes begin sessions to resolve one issue in their lives but eventually come to understand that there are layers to their pain, some layers that don't even belong to them but rather to people in their family and lineage. You yourself may have started off thinking your struggles were caused by one thing, and only later come to the realization that what you've been struggling with is inherited trauma. When trauma is passed down, it can look like other symptoms, such as chronic depression, crippling anxiety, and lack of focus, so it can at first be difficult to spot.

The good thing here is that you've recognized that there's an inherited nature to your pain, and so now you can do something about it. That realization is critical for the work ahead, but it's also a lot to come to terms with, so it's natural if your heart feels heavy as you enter this healing quest. As you work, your heart will sometimes soften and at other times get even heavier. It's important to bear in mind that your healing won't be linear. There will be waves of emotions. There will be high-highs and low-lows. Setting your expectations for the journey ahead can be useful in helping you flow through the experience. It will be critical in helping you prepare for the hard moments ahead.

Anytime you engage in depth work, there is always the chance that you'll experience an elevation in your stress levels. Opening these doors psychologically can be triggering. Therefore, it is imperative for you to have a coping plan in place for the entirety of your work here. It's also essential because as the body is triggered, it kicks the nervous system into a sympathetic response. Essentially, your emotions might force your body into survival mode. When your body is in survival mode, all nonessential functions, including the complex thinking that you'll need to relieve your stress, will be compromised.

Emotional outbursts, or the experience of emotions becoming over-whelming and pouring out, require that a person always have a road map for how to cope with difficult emotions. This road map allows a person to have preplanned coping skills in place for when their emotional journey feels like too much. It will prepare you for any experience that produces distress, increase your chances of being able to help yourself through your emotional response, and help you lift yourself out of survival mode more quickly. To initiate a cope-ahead plan, please consider the following steps:

- Choose a quiet, comfortable spot where you aren't likely to be interrupted.
- Decide on one grounding method that can help you come back to your body. One I find to be helpful is grounding with the five senses. To do this, you list things you notice around you while seated in place. You start by looking around and listing five things you can see. Then you scan the room again and list four things you can touch. After you're done with the sense of touch, you move into listing three things you can hear. After you've finished that list, you look around again for two things you can smell. Finally, you list one thing that you can taste.
- After you're done grounding yourself, you can move into a cope-ahead practice, where you imagine surviving a tough scenario.
- Start by imagining a situation where you're likely to feel *mildly* triggered. Take your time to imagine this as vividly as possible.

- Rehearse in your mind coping through the situation. What this means is that you literally envision yourself finding a solution to the problem and coming out of it feeling well.
- Now take ten deep, slow breaths, inhaling for 5 seconds and exhaling for 7 seconds, while continuing to imagine yourself feeling well and at ease.
- Finally, allow yourself a moment of respite. You can do this by just sitting in place for a few more seconds.

This practice allows you to see one primary thing: every problem is survivable. You can find a solution and move forward. You can come back to this exercise whenever the work ahead feels like an impossible task and remind yourself that this, too, is survivable.

A Gentle Reminder

Intergenerational healing requires you to feel like the work is safe and tolerable. So go at your own pace and notice when you need to take a break. If this work starts to feel like it's just too much to do on your own, seek a co-healing partner or a trauma-responsive mental health professional to help guide you through this deep work.

Sound Baths to Keep You Grounded

It is my intention that you feel as psychologically safe as possible as you read this book and engage in its practices. But what is psychological safety? It's your capacity to feel yourself in the present without the need to run away, either physically or mentally. If you feel safe, you can stay in the present and follow through on the healing methods I propose. And so, to that end, I would like to introduce a practice to help you anchor yourself: sound bath meditations. And just in case you're unfamiliar with what a sound bath is, let me briefly explain.

Sound medicine refers to the use of sound and, specifically, sound waves at certain frequencies, to create vibrations in the body that can help the body feel ease and healing. Sound baths emit vibrational frequencies that work at the cellular level. And it is this sound energy that recalibrates whatever tension is blocked or frozen in the nervous system. It's almost like the vibrations are gently shaking the body's energy back into place. So when your nervous system is taken out of balance due to high-level stress and trauma, sound waves have a way, at a very granular, cellular level, of helping move it back into balance. And when trauma is a part of our daily lives, we need to keep the idea of balance at the center, or risk getting thrown off-kilter.

Sound baths have a long history, predating modern medicine by centuries. Quartz singing bowls, my chosen instrument for sound healing, have their origins in Tibetan Buddhist practices. When struck, the bowls emit multiple notes that can help remove blocked energy by creating a vibration in specific areas of your body, also known as chakra centers. These practices have been around for well over two thousand years and are traditionally accompanied by meditation and chanting. The practice of chanting has ancestral roots in places across the world, and when matched with other healing sounds, it can produce an almost immediate calming effect in a person's mind and body.

It is my goal to equip you with as many tools as I can to help keep you in a state of balance. The more tools you have, the more you will feel emotionally steady. In an effort to help ground you, promote your healing, and connect you to ancestral wisdom, I have borrowed from this ancient practice and produced three sound bath meditations, one to accompany each section of this book. In borrowing said practices, I would like for both you and me to honor their origins, the people of Tibet and their descendants, who have used this method of sound as a practice well before you and I ever inhabited Earth, and its original purpose of communal healing.

Each sound bath that accompanies this book is meant to deepen your experience. If you can, welcome these sound baths as the wrap-up to each section and allow yourself a moment of respite and rest while you listen.

See appendix D for your healing sound bath meditations.

Healing in Community

Tackling all this alone might seem daunting. If it leaves you feeling like you need community, a useful strategy for healing is to bring another person on this journey with you. Healing with people you consider to be an essential part of your community can be beneficial to your healing journey. But remember, regardless of whether you choose to heal with a partner or heal your own soul, it is your choice and it is one that you will intuitively know is the right or wrong one for you.

If you have decided to follow this book with someone, bring that fellow cycle breaker to mind. It can be an ancestor, or it can be a living person you invite to actually do this work with you, step-by-step, chapter-by-chapter. Critically, if you invite in a living person, they must be equally committed to doing the hard work of breaking cycles and in helping support you as you break yours.

Whenever I propose this to clients, I typically sense some hesitation. If that's how you're feeling, I don't blame you. My clients usually think I am asking them to invite their family members on their healing journey. That the ones with the deepest emotional pain should do this work with them. That couldn't be further from my intention. Instead, I ask you to consider working with someone (family or not, living or in the spirit world) who contributes to your psychological safety, as opposed to someone who might trigger you. It makes more sense to work with someone who helps you feel safe when the work is so emotionally demanding. I'm not asking you to take on more of an emotional burden but instead offering a way to alleviate some of the burden you already carry. If the concept of co-healing, or healing in community, is appealing to you, this is your opportunity to consider who that person will be. If someone comes to mind, invite them on this journey. If you feel that your healing will be greater if you continue this process on your own, listen to that intuition. Whichever path you choose, be sure to grab your writing materials to enter into your first cycle-breaking practice.

Breaking the Cycle: Break Your Generational Agreement

Until now, a part of you has held an unconscious agreement to show up as a wounded self and keep the old patterns that have held your lineage in pain and trauma. This agreement has maintained the cycle. But stepping out as a cycle breaker requires breaking this agreement. It requires a release. You will have to commit to letting go of old patterns and welcoming in healthier ones. So, in order to do this, I would like to help you break that old contract and write a new one. Grab a separate sheet of paper for this exercise, and write your version of the following:

- Since [enter your own date], I have been operating as a wounded self. I have unconsciously fed into an intergenerational trauma cycle that has kept me in decades of hurt. Sometimes without my own conscious knowing that it was doing this, it has stunted my life and that of my lineage. I no longer wish to be bound to this contract. I release it and let it go.
- Now take the contract and rip it to shreds.

- Now write a new contract in your designated journal that helps you enter into an agreement to commit to the cycle-breaking journey. You can write a version of the following:
  - Starting [enter today's date], I will be wholeheartedly stepping into the identity of cycle breaker. I will consciously feed my life and those around me from an elevated multigenerational and ancestral consciousness. I will do this for myself, my lineage, and my collective.
- Sign and date your contract.
- Reflect on how this practice was for you. How did you feel it in your mind, body, and spirit? That is, how did you feel it in your soul?

What You've Learned So Far

In this chapter, we began to acknowledge what brings you into reading *Break the Cycle*: the fact that you are a cycle breaker. We defined what a cycle breaker is and left some room for you to also add to that definition. You also learned how to set up your healing for the chapters ahead, and we ended this chapter with an invitation to break the cycle by breaking the subconscious contract you have had to a lineage of pain. This is major. I hope you're proud. Your ancestors surely are. Now let's continue working through some reflection questions.

REFLECTION QUESTIONS

How does it feel to apply the concept of cycle breaker to yourself?
How are you feeling about the setup for the work ahead?
How was it for you to break the contract with your past cycles?

CHAPTER 2

Your Intergenerational Higher Self

you are one person
but when you move
an entire community
walks through you
you go nowhere alone

—Rupi Kaur

Now that you know you're a cycle breaker, it's time to take the next step forward to understand your *intergenerational higher self.* Getting in touch with your intergenerational higher self requires that you acknowledge and access the resilience and ancestral wisdom you already hold within you. Oftentimes, when approaching the intergenerational healing journey, people want to get straight to what's hurting. This makes it easy to lose sight of an equally important aspect of this experience, your intergenerational resilience. Trauma isn't the only experience that can be passed down from generation to generation. There may have been gentle words of love, power, or affirmation that were reflected to you as well. Understanding how to approach your intergenerational healing first requires that you connect with your intergenerational wisdom. It is there that you will find strength and inner knowledge to help you acquire stamina for the road ahead. And although it is already an inherited trait that you have, I would like to further orient you on how you can tap into your generational resilience.

You might have heard of the concept of the *higher self*. Your higher self is the version of you that has experienced a transformation through healing. It is a version of you that's no longer neck-deep in trauma. The higher self is not a perfectly healed self, because perfect healing is a myth. Instead, it's your higher consciousness. It's where your wisest mind lies. It is where a lot of your innate wisdom lives. It's the version of you that feels grounded and not emotionally shaky. It's how you feel when you have a clear and steady mind. Your intergenerational higher self is all these things and more. It's a reflection of both your own innate wisdom *and* your ancestral wisdom. It's both the innate knowledge that you hold *and* the knowledge that was passed down. It's a layered higher self. An intergenerational higher self is the living embodiment of intergenerational abundance. Honoring your intergenerational higher self means living in alignment with a higher purpose. It's about redirecting the energy you would have used for self-destruction and shifting it toward intergenerational elevation. Here, we'll aim to get you in touch with this intergenerational higher self and its wisdom by first helping you understand it better, then helping you access it.

First, let me offer an example from my own life—the moment I finally stepped into my own intergenerational higher self. My mother shared a powerful set of words with me during the first semester of my doctoral studies. I was facing the worst impostor syndrome of my life. Being a Black Latina immigrant from a working-class background in an Ivy League institution meant that I was constantly confronted with reminders of how much I didn't belong. I was made to feel that way through a constant barrage of race- and class-motivated abuse that I faced almost daily. When I told my mother about these experiences and how much I wanted to quit my program—the racism and classism were nearly unbearable—she echoed some words of generational wisdom that I never forgot. She said, "You come from a lineage of strong and resourceful people. God has your back and so do we. You are already victorious. Now go back in there and show them how powerful you are." And that's exactly what I did. I stood in my generational power and my generational wisdom. I showed up as my intergenerational higher self. Every time I would feel impostor syndrome creating fear in me, I would remember my mother's words, "You are powerful," and I would say these words out loud. And it was true. The impostor syndrome that comes from generations of my communities being told that they don't belong had crept into my soul. My mother's words, however, reminded me to break up with that generational lie. I was a woman from a lineage of power, resourcefulness, strength, resilience, and wisdom. I now know that impostor syndrome is not my truth but an inheritance from generations of being marginalized. It's a way in which I and many others in my communities have been isolated, shut out, and made to feel like we don't belong. But we do belong and I stepped wholeheartedly into that truth. My intergenerational higher self grew out of this moment. It helped me through one of the toughest moments in my life, and I hope it can do the same for you.

How the Higher Self Becomes Intergenerational

Your higher self is a place of self-enlightenment. It's the wisest piece of your mind. All your truest desires for yourself and for your healing are captured in your higher self. Those flashes of intuition, inspiration, and nonverbal communication are all part of this internal experience. Your intergenerational higher self is a place of both self-enlightenment *and* ancestral enlightenment. Your ancestors' cumulative intentions, wishes, and wisdom are layered on top of your own, to contribute to your intergenerational higher self. When you're attuned to your intergenerational higher self, you're in a place that is loving, nurturing, ancestrally wise, and intuitive. It is sacred in that way. When you tap into this generational elevation, you are able to experience greater calm, trust in yourself, curiosity, and self-awareness. It enlightens and fulfills you through these gifts.

Intergenerational trauma forces us to numb our creativity, joy, and overall zest for life. Your intergenerational higher self, however, helps you reignite your potential and rise out of the ashes. When you continually commit to reprogramming your soul, your new default will be to lean on your internal wisdom. Eventually, you will automatically use this tool more than your current coping mechanisms, which will allow you to rewire your brain and nervous system to experience greater ease in the face of stress. There are many ways in which you can start the process of connecting to your intergenerational higher self. Let's highlight some that you can start with.

Tapping Into Your Intergenerational Higher Self

Your intergenerational higher self is a tool, an instrument of healing, a catalyst for generational liberation. Tapping into it means you are using the innate tools locked within you to help alleviate the pain that has been passed down. And there are both passive and active ways to do this. For some people, an intergenerational higher self comes into contact with them first. This future version of themselves shows them symbols, signs, ideas, dreams, and stories that they didn't know they had access to. This wisdom might feel otherworldly. And yet, since these messages come from a place deep within, they will feel grounded, sturdy, trustworthy. Here are some ways your intergenerational higher self might be trying to reach you, so pay attention:

- **While Sitting in Silence**—Silence is the breeding ground for our most burrowed points of insight. Find a quiet place to sit and focus on your immediate surroundings. Listen to where your thoughts go. If your mind wanders, that's OK. Just gently bring it back to focus. This present-tense orientation can help you experience moments more mindfully and clear out the clutter of your mind for the messages that are hoping to make their way from your subconscious mind into your conscious mind.

- **Through Active Meditation**—If your mind is more focused inward, you will find it easier to turn your attention toward your intergenerational higher self's messages and guidance. A simple sitting meditation can help you get closer to what your elevated consciousness is hoping you can hear. But if you're someone whose mind is extra busy, you can also move your body as a form of meditation. Some people choose to go on walks without their phones and take in the sounds and signs around them. A gentle walk can help you enter a different state of consciousness, because it offers a powerful mindful moment for you to connect to that wiser part of you much easier. If a walking meditation isn't something you're interested in, some alternatives could be yoga, tai chi, and dance.

- **When Dreaming**—Your sleep state of dreaming is out of your conscious control, and in it, your mind is able to tap into greater depths of your subconscious. Your dreams are able to offer you higher-level messages, should you be willing to listen. Some of the older, more psychoanalytic fields of psychotherapy include dream analysis to evaluate deep, complex traumas. Dreams send us messages about our emotional world. Taking heed of your dreams is a good way to measure and track where our unconscious mind lingers.

- **While Getting Out into Nature**—Connecting with the natural elements is not only nourishing to the soul but can also help us connect with the many little miracles that exist around us. Earth is truly wise and ancestral. Tapping into the different layers of nature can help us capture wisdom that is right in front of us. The task here can be as simple as walking barefoot on grass or foraging in your local park or green space. You can be as creative as you wish when getting curious about Earth's little wonders.

- **While Having a Dialogue with Your Wiser Self**—Having ongoing conversations with your intergenerational higher self, as if they were an actual person in front of you, may help you tap into any information that your intergenerational higher self is hoping for you to know. For some people, it helps to look in the mirror and literally talk with themselves. This can get you into the practice of having a chat with yourself on an ongoing basis. You'll be surprised at what comes up when you befriend your intergenerational higher self in this way.

- **Through Letters and Journal Entries**—I like to think of writing letters or journal entries as written meditations. You're placing your thoughts, desires, fantasies, questions, and intuitions onto paper. This way, you may be able to focus more concretely on what questions you're seeking answers to and return to them later. Write a few notes in your journal and see what aspects of your intergenerational wisdom come up.

- **Through Imagery Exercises**—Visualization can harness the power of a wiser self-connection in a multitude of ways. Imagining your intergenerational higher self coming to you with a healing word is a powerful tool. This tool gives you an immersive experience of safety and containment. Let's try it now:

  - Think of your intergenerational higher self and see if an image comes to mind. How are they dressed? What's their posture? How do they speak? Do they look like you in a different era of life? Do they instead look like someone else, perhaps a guide or an ancestor? Are they in a human or more mythical, spiritual form? Get curious about them and use your creativity.

- Then, connect with them and listen to their words. It can oftentimes help to journal about these exercises to keep a log of what you heard and saw.

What comes up for every person as a result of these exercises will be individual, and many if not all of these practices will be new to you, so an important rule of thumb is to be open and receptive to whatever you feel. The ways that messages come to you may feel unnatural at first, but remember that with openings for greater consciousness, we receive bigger and more direct messages. So, every time you practice, be curious about what messages are being left for you and how you can open your mind to receive them. There can be so many benefits to receiving wiser thoughts, including:

- Getting a new perspective that could help guide you
- Helping you feel more grounded
- Increasing your capacity to surrender to the wisdom of your intergenerational higher self
- Helping you grow in greater appreciation for your own innate wisdom
- Helping you develop patience and perhaps even self-compassion and collective compassion
- Helping you understand just how interconnected you are with the elements of life and the universe
- Helping you embrace the multiple layers of who you are and where you come from
- Helping you hold on to hope, despite having lived a life that has disrupted your sense of hope

The message here is that there are many ways in which these practices could add depth to your journey. Lean into them, even if they feel new and out of the norm of how you typically tap into your wisdom.

Remember, this is about elevating that wisdom and increasing the ways in which you can be resilient. These exercises can help.

Breaking the Cycle: Stepping Into Your Intergenerational Higher Self

I'd like to introduce you to a modified version of an intervention we have in psychology called the empty chair technique. This technique derives from a type of psychoanalytic psychotherapy called Gestalt therapy, which aims to see a whole person as the sum of different parts. It helps us look at situations from multiple perspectives, in order to see how they are all interconnected. The original empty chair technique involves one empty chair. The one I created for the intergenerational process requires three chairs placed side-by-side. One chair will symbolize your wounded self, one will symbolize your intergenerational higher self, and one will symbolize your intergenerational ancestral self. The intergenerational higher self reflects all the qualities we have discussed throughout this chapter. And the wounded self signifies the part of you that carries the wound of intergenerational trauma, while the intergenerational ancestral self refers to the part of you that holds your wisest point of insight and ancestral wisdom.

A note to consider about this practice: if mobility to different chairs is not accessible to you, you can envision yourself in the different chairs as you navigate this exercise. Another modification that can be added is to think of the words and affirmations you can speak to yourself, rather than speaking them out loud.

- Start by sitting in the chair you have designated as the wounded self chair.
- If it feels safe, close your eyes to enhance your focus.
- Now consider these questions:

- ▪ What feels wounded?
- ▪ What emotions come up as you think about this wound?
- ▪ What do you feel in your body?
- ▪ How has your spirit captured this wound?
- ▪ What do you wish you could hear in this moment?
- Take a few deep breaths as you sit in this experience.
- Now open your eyes and move to the intergenerational higher self chair.
- Turn toward the wounded self chair.
- See if you can envision your wounded self sitting there.
- Bring to mind something that you wish to say to your wounded self. What does your wounded self need to hear right now?
- Now say out loud what you believe your wounded self needs to hear.
- Now sit on the intergenerational ancestral self chair.
- Turn again toward the wounded self chair.
- Continue to envision your wounded self sitting there.
- Bring to mind something that you believe your ancestors would say to your wounded self. What ancestral message does your wounded self need to hear right now?
- Now say out loud what you believe your wounded self could hear, from an ancestral point of view.
- And now, still in your ancestral chair, turn to your intergenerational higher self chair.
- Envision your intergenerational higher self sitting there.
- Bring to mind something that you wish to say to your intergenerational higher self from an ancestral point of view.
- Now say out loud what you believe your intergenerational higher self needs to hear from an ancestral point of view.
- Close your eyes and envision all three parts of you coming together as one integrated whole.
- Take in the experience for as long as is needed.

- Take a few breaths to transition out of your practice.
- When you're ready, write a few lines in your journal about your experience.

What You've Learned So Far

In this chapter, you learned all about your intergenerational higher self, the part of you that is infinitely wise and carries ancestral wisdom. You were guided through ways to tap into this generational resilience and were taken through an intergenerational empty chair exercise to further connect you to your generational insight. Take a look at the reflection questions that follow and write whatever comes to mind in response to them, before transitioning to the next chapter, where we will focus on unpacking how intergenerational trauma gets processed as body memory.

REFLECTION QUESTIONS

What's it like for you to envision yourself as an intergenerational higher self?

How was it for you to engage in the intergenerational empty chair technique?

How else would you like to show up as your healed self in the context of intergenerational work?

CHAPTER 3

Your Body Remembers Your Trauma

Trauma is not just an event that took place sometime in the past; it is also the imprint left by that experience on mind, brain, and body.

—Bessel van der Kolk

When our bodies get weighed down by toxic stress, when they experience strain over and over, they can start to wear down. We all have a neurological wear-and-tear meter that neuroscientists call the *allostatic load*. The allostatic load is the cumulative burden of chronic stress that the body accumulates over time. When stress piles up without enough nervous system rest and repair, it overwhelms our allostatic load. This depletes the body's capacity to find its own balance, and as a result, it compromises the body's capacity to stay healthy. As you might imagine, this is incredibly important to consider for those of us suffering from intergenerational strain, because our bodies and our ancestors' bodies have been in an allostatic overload for generations. This is a lot to take in, so go gently as you read further.

Emotional trauma can cause physical bodily damage. Inflamed minds yield inflamed bodies. Several dysfunctions of the body's neuro-

36

logical and immune functions can be mapped back to the psychological wear and tear we place on the body. People with excessive emotional trauma—those who are prone to have inadvertently overextended their own allostatic capacities—can have livers that overproduce glucocorticoid, for example. This can then impact both liver function and, interestingly enough, the main memory centers of your brain. Another example of this is how trauma triggers the overreactive trimming or "pruning" of your neurons that can happen as a result of longstanding stress, which can place you at risk for neurological degeneration, the kind that can trigger conditions like Lou Gehrig's disease (ALS). Chronic stress inflames your body in innumerable ways. And when your genes start recording all of this hyperinflammatory activity for an extended period of time, epigenetic changes occur. But that isn't where the story ends. You can rebalance your body to reduce your risk for physical health complications or reduce the progression of diseases that have inhabited your body. One way you can start doing this is by helping your nervous system relax more and release the overburden of inflammation situated in your body. You've been doing this with some of the practices in this book, so you're already ahead, but let's continue to learn more about the mind-body connection and additional ways to help relieve your body of toxic stress.

The Mind and Body Are One

An estimated 60 to 80 percent of primary care visits are the result of an underlying stress-related reason. I hope I have sent you on enough mental loops to cement the core message here: the mind and body are inextricably linked, and stress impacts both. Conversely, when you take care of your mind, your body will feel that care. If you're releasing emotional heaviness from your mind through healing work, your body will feel lighter and less tense. Mind relaxation exercises help heal your body, and body relaxation exercises help heal your mind. The two work together in a health-promoting cycle, working to achieve balance for you at all times.

Examples of this connection can be found throughout your body. When your nervous system is relaxed, you are more able to achieve clarity of mind and perform complex thinking, and your problem-solving skills are enhanced. This is all because your body isn't in survival mode, and so your cortical brain, which is responsible for higher-level thinking, has the capacity to achieve optimal functioning. Another example of this mind-body relationship is found in your gut microbiome, where many of your neurotransmitters, the chemicals that help balance your mood, are housed. When you eat meals that nourish your gut microbiome, neurochemicals like serotonin, GABA, dopamine, acetylcholine, norepinephrine, and melatonin are impacted as well. A well-regulated mood, in turn, can help improve digestion, energy levels, sleep quality, and overall body balance. The mind and body are made to coexist in a collaborative relationship that's supposed to work to keep you healthy.

Trauma, however, can disrupt this balancing system and spiral the mind-body cycle in the opposite direction. Emotional pain affects your body negatively, which in turn impacts your mental health. A part of what has kept generations of families in this downward mind-body spiral is that, in many societies, the medical system fails to treat the mind and body together.

Traditionally, Western medical science treats the mind and body as two systems that operate apart from one another. We don't help people relieve stress as a way to improve their physical health, but we should. Under the current medical model, each organ is treated independently, rather than being viewed as an interactive global system. A cardiologist treats your heart, a gastroenterologist will treat your digestive tract, a pulmonologist will focus on your lungs, a neurologist will focus on the brain, and so on. But there aren't specialties that focus on identifying how stress factors have led the heart to have structural complications;

or how a toxic relationship has made your stomach turn chronically, causing what feels like irritable bowel syndrome; or how grief is directed at the lungs and that chronic shortness of breath can be a trauma response related to complicated grief; or how your brain's neurons prune away and decrease in volume with chronic stress, leaving you vulnerable to neurodegenerative disease. Your mind and body are a single system, not two independent ones. So a whole-person medical approach, like the one you find in this book, that is holistic and accounts for how the mind and body work as a unit, is essential for sustainable healing.

The more that you are able to see how your emotional life is a body-centered experience, the more you will see how critical it is to integrate the body into the healing of generational pain. If it feels like a lot to wrap your head around, I understand. It took some time for me to get it, too, but let me explain how I arrived at this understanding.

During my doctoral training, I was chosen for a holistic mental health clinical fellowship, designated by a grant from the US Department of Health and Human Services and in collaboration with Columbia University Irving Medical Center. I held multiple roles throughout my three-year fellowship. In my first year, my fellowship director, Dr. Elizabeth Fraga, assigned me the role of program coordinator, where I got to work on the development of a pilot program that would place me in different medical specialty clinics across the Columbia hospital system. Our aim was to help patients who were suffering from comorbid conditions, meaning that they were struggling with both mental and physical health complications. We designed the program around the mainly Latine community of Washington Heights in Upper Manhattan, where the Columbia Medical Center campus occupies land. Once the program had been conceptualized and its integration into the medical center was complete, my role was to provide holistic psychological services in Spanish to community members who qualified with the clinical conditions we sought to service. Among the mental health symptoms that were being treated were depression, anxiety, panic disorder, bipolar disorder, post-traumatic stress disorder (PTSD), attention deficit hyperactivity disorder (ADHD), and psychosis. Physical health symptoms that we worked with were cardiac problems, lung conditions, autoimmune conditions, stomach issues, neurological disorders, and peri- and postpartum complications.

During the second year, I was placed as the mental health clinician in several specialty clinics throughout the hospital (e.g., cardiology, neurology, gynecology, and primary care offices). My clinical task was to offer mental health services to patients who came in with physical complaints where no obvious physical cause could be found, or those who had comorbid physical and psychiatric conditions that were suspected to be linked. Additionally, I trained other hospital clinicians (e.g., physicians, nurses, social workers, and clinical assistants) on the underlying mental health conditions frequently behind the physical health complaints that our patients came in with. We worked as a team. We shared patients, shared ideas, shared sessions, and were working as a mind- *and* body-centered team of clinicians. We were integrating ancient healing practices into this supermodern medical system. It was truly innovative and, for many of our patients, validating and healing. It was a community-centered and people-centered psychology model that aimed to relieve the ailments that plagued our community members, not keep them as perpetual patients.

At one point, one of my clinical supervisors and the then clinic director, Dr. Diana Puñales-Morejón, wanted to bring Spanish-speaking spiritualists to the clinic's team meetings to train staff on the ways we could more effectively integrate ancient cultural-spiritual understandings into our work. We understood that the work we needed to do in our community would require a holistic mind-body-spirit lens that was culturally relevant and responsible.

We were working to build the future of health care, an integrated model of medicine. I remember the sense of duty I felt to do this well.

This was my community, after all. My family lived so close to the campus that once, when I was in the gynecology clinic lobby looking for one of my patients, I heard my pregnant cousin scream from across the room, "Mariel, hey!" I froze for a moment, because traditional psychology tells us that we are supposed to be these blank slates with no personal connection to the work and the people we serve. So the next day, in my supervision session, I nervously told Dr. Puñales-Morejón and Dr. Santos Vales (my other supervisor) that I had run into my cousin in the lobby, believing that I could possibly be told to not interact with community members outside the treatment room. Instead, they had a good laugh about it. They knew it was my moment of initiation into community healing work. Dr. Puñales-Morejón said half-jokingly, "Welcome to community psychology!" and Dr. Vales said agreeably, "These are our people we're helping." In that moment, I had a monumental realization. We were in a community that was our own, doing holistic community work that was rooted in how our communities have healed for centuries. This work was both personal and professional. We were profoundly devoted to providing the best care to our beloved people. We understood that we needed to think beyond the traditional models of psychotherapy and step into models that actually work for the long term. When we saw how many people in the hospital came to us with generational histories of pain, comorbid conditions, and stress-derived physical symptoms, we understood that the soundest and most ethical model of care was a holistic model that honored the mind, body, and spirit of the people we were commissioned to serve. That is when we truly started seeing global change in our patients. That is the model I am committed to teaching you in the pages of this book.

At this moment you're likely wondering, What does it look like to be healing in this more global way? The quick answer to that is, you're already doing holistic healing through the practices you're learning in this book. Each of the Breaking the Cycle practices targets at least one aspect of the mind or body and almost all have a spiritual undertone. I've taken your whole soul into account with each practice. So if the idea of stress being in the body sounds daunting to approach, start with understanding that you already have tools at your disposal; just flip back through the exercises in this book. You can repeat these practices time and again until you start seeing tangible results. That's what I have done with my clients, repeated these practices until we saw improvement. Let's go into the stories of Nola, a patient whose pain was deeply embedded in her body, and of my sister Lady's own journey of mind-body pain to help illustrate this holistic approach some more.

Grief Is in the Lungs

Nola had a chronic lung condition. She didn't smoke, didn't work in hazardous conditions, and didn't do anything else that could have normally caused a condition like hers. On any given day, breathing would simply become harder for her. This happened enough times that she was eventually diagnosed with idiopathic chronic lung disease. *Idiopathic* meaning that it sprouted spontaneously with no known cause. Over the years, she underwent several interventions, including surgical biopsies where a doctor excised her lung tissue in search of answers to this mystery inflammation. And her doctors kept attending to the physical lung while ignoring her troubles of the mind and spirit. Her treatment did not account for the layers of stress this woman was under or the pervasive function of intergenerational stress-based inflammation contributing to her reduced organ function.

Once I started working with Nola, I looped in our clinic nutritionist, social worker, and physicians to devise a holistic plan that could help release some of the stress factors in her life. If we couldn't take away her lung inflammation altogether, at least we could limit its progression. When she came to my sessions, we worked on holistic mental health methods (i.e., all the practices you have at your disposal through this book already, like deep breathing and visualization, ventral vagal stimulation exercises, meditations, other body sensory practices, and, of course, talking through her intergenerational traumas). I attended her sessions with her nutritionist and physician to offer my input and learn about their recommendations on health-promoting and mood-balancing nutrition. Our social worker got her connected to a clinical trial where she could receive cutting-edge monitoring of her lung function. And most important, all her doctors and specialists were connecting about hormone levels, lifestyle changes, disease analysis, and healing progress. We worked together to bring Nola's health up to an optimal level. And it did help. With time, she was managing to breathe better, get more active, and feel emotionally lighter under our care.

But for me, Nola's case was more than professional. It was personal. While I was treating Nola, I was also caring for my sister, Lady. A few years prior, she, too, had developed lung disease. Hers, however, was a consequence of an inflammatory condition called rheumatoid arthritis. Her lungs became the primary source of her arthritic inflammation. As the eldest sibling, my sister had always had a lot of pressure placed upon her. It's a common practice in Latine homes to assign undue responsibility to the eldest daughter, especially a first-generation immigrant daughter. It's a cultural practice that can have devastating consequences on children, giving them too great a responsibility at too young an age. She has always been the one to go to. She spent her life taking care of everyone. Not just me, but oftentimes our parents as well. Along with this chronic sense of familial responsibility, she experienced other traumas, including poverty and my father's absence when he was separated from us for ten years while waiting for his US green card. A lifetime of carrying everyone's emotional weight was now being expressed in her physical body. The condition nearly cost her her life.

I think my sister, like Nola, held on to a lot of grief. In particular, the grief of a lost childhood. A childhood sacrificed in service of making my family's "American dream" come true and taking care of my parents and me. Now, my sister and I look back and talk about how she was parentified, which is when parents give a child some responsibilities that belong to a parent, like partly caring for their younger siblings. For most of our childhood, my sister was tasked with caring for me, while our mom worked two jobs. When my sister got sick, suddenly the roles were reversed and I was the one taking care of her. I functioned as a doctoral student by day and my sister's nurse by night. Sometimes I'd sleep in a hospital recliner at her bedside, then hop on the train from the Bronx to Upper Manhattan to see my clients, head downtown to supervision with my holistic mental health supervisor, Dr. Traci Stein, trek back uptown to attend classes in the afternoon, transition to teaching my own classes at Columbia's main campus in Morningside Heights, then shoot back up to Washington Heights to teach at the Columbia Medical Center's Genetic Counseling department, and finally head back up to the Bronx to my hospital recliner. Phew!

Going through it, I didn't think anything of it. I didn't have time to. I had a duty to help my sister survive, and I had a drive to finish this degree to help more people heal. I think generational resilience carried me through those times. I was able to still get good grades and soaked up every bit of holistic knowledge that I could, because not only did my patients depend on me, but now my sister did too.

What I learned in that time I applied to all aspects of my life. When I learned about the implications of inflammation on the body at my fellowship, I would share that information with my colleagues *and* with my sister. When I learned about the benefits of practicing holistic meditation, I brought it back to my patients *and* to my family. I started practicing tai chi and yoga. And guess who joined me? That's right: my patients *and* my sister started practicing tai chi and yoga too. In class, I learned about the implications of the gut microbiome on mood and health, and I brought that information to my patients and my sister.

Whatever knowledge I obtained about holistic care went back to the community and back into my personal spaces. My sister experienced a positive spike in her lung function. It actually started slightly improving in a short amount of time. Unfortunately, by the time we started integrating these body-centered practices, my sister's lungs were barely functional at all, and a slight improvement wasn't nearly enough to keep her alive. She was already on oxygen 24-7 and needed a transplant as soon as possible. We were fortunate for our organ donor's selfless act to provide my sister with the opportunity for a transplant and the second chance at life that she received as a result. But we never abandoned the lessons we learned about the mind and body. And we continue to practice holistic healing to this day.

I do still wish I had learned about holistically treating trauma earlier. I wish I had understood that for centuries, in Eastern cultures, it has been understood that grief is captured in the lungs, in the heart chakra. I wish I had known how the body attacks itself when it's too inflamed by stress and why anti-inflammatory mind-body practices are critical to healing. I wish I had been aware of a whole world of ancient healing wisdom, and what it had to teach me about bringing balance to the body before the body gives up. I wish that we hadn't suffered such a deep disconnection from ancestral healing in the modern world and that we wouldn't have to work so hard to gain this wisdom back at such critical moments, when the pain we carry threatens our life. And most of all, I wish that for both my patients and my sister, there could have been preventative methods that might have shielded them from a traumatizing set of medical procedures. I wish I could've saved everyone from their grief. I wish I could have saved myself from my own suffering.

But I couldn't. I had to accept that I couldn't. All I could do was educate myself, my clients, my family, my community, and now all of you. I can't undo the past, but I can help equip you with knowledge and help you build a life that's more balanced, now and for generations. For

my sister, breaking the cycle meant reconnecting to her body holistically. It also meant that as an eldest daughter of immigrants, she had to
abandon the burden of saving everyone, because now she was the one
that needed saving. She had to unlearn her trauma response, which was
people-pleasing with a heavy dose of guilt. And it meant that she
needed to grieve the childhood that she was never allowed to have. In
order to live a fuller life, she had to drop the emotional baggage that
weighed her lungs down. You will also have to relinquish the weight of
stress that is planting itself in you. Let's dive into more of that stress-
based knowledge that can be helpful along your journey. Remember to
breathe deeply and take gentle pauses as you continue reading.

The Generational Impact of Stress

Stress-influenced chronic disease can run through generations of families. This is particularly true of inflammatory diseases (e.g., autoimmune
disorders, cardiac diseases, and gastrointestinal issues). Exposure to
adverse childhood experiences (ACEs) has been associated with chronic
inflammation and an elevated risk for inflammatory responses in the
body. Children living with adverse histories tend to be more defense-
less against recurring infections and more susceptible to chronic inflammatory conditions, such as heart conditions, arthritis, diabetes,
depression, gastrointestinal conditions, different cancers, autoimmune
disorders, dementia, and other ailments throughout their entire lives.
Heart disease and other chronic illnesses that persist into adulthood
have been linked to psychological abuse suffered early in life. One study
that focused on people living with systemic lupus found a common history of emotional deprivation in childhood, showing a correlation between presence of the disease and a fractured relationship with caregivers.

Long-term studies looking at how children view their parents (e.g.,
positively and warm, or negatively and cold) related the elevated risk for

heart disease and hypertension to those who viewed their parents or caregivers with less warmth. And one Harvard and Johns Hopkins study even found that people who reported having less warm and loving relationships growing up were more likely to develop cancer in midlife. The stress-disease connection is real, and it is harmful to the body's equilibrium.

Unaddressed intergenerational stress can make it almost impossible for the body to achieve balance (homeostasis). In severe cases, trauma might destroy the body's capacity to stay alive, because it either aggravates existing health issues or creates new diseases in your body. Take, for example, one muscle group that is strongly affected by tension in the body: the heart. Stress hormones like adrenaline, noradrenaline, and cortisol are highly responsible for inflammation in the circulatory system, and especially the coronary arteries, which are the pathways to stress-induced heart attacks. And where there's inflammation chronically directed at an organ, the immune system's function is usually suppressed, leaving room for an elevated risk for infection and other diseases. I'll illustrate a few other examples of common stress-disease connections, but before we go there, let's do a gentle pause, because you're taking in a lot of heavy information.

Do a quick body scan and notice how your body is taking in this body-centered information. Are your muscles tensing up or more relaxed? Are there any sensations that you didn't notice before? If so, shift your attention to the place where you're experiencing any sensation. If your hands can reach that area, give yourself a gentle massage or simply tap the area lightly. Increase the depth of your breath by breathing in for more seconds and breathing out for more seconds. And when you're ready, let's look at a few more examples.

Another major example of this mind-body connection is the depression that runs through families. Depression is a leading cause of disability worldwide. Cases of depression have surpassed cancer, HIV/AIDS, and cardiovascular and respiratory diseases combined.

Depression is not just a mental illness, but a bodily one too. It can be so hard for people to get their bodies moving when they're depressed. That's why you oftentimes hear that people who are depressed have the energy only to stay in bed or on a couch all day. That's partly because depression itself has an inflammatory function, meaning the depressed brain and body are inflamed. This may explain why some antidepressants don't work for certain people. The function of some antidepressants is to trigger or inhibit certain neurotransmitters responsible for mood; however, this line of treatment does not address depression's inflammatory process, which is critical to account for.

Stress can also have a direct impact on sex organs and reproduction. Excess amounts of cortisol can impact the biochemical functioning of sex organs by creating imbalances in hormone levels, which interfere with sperm production and contribute to impotence, abnormal menses, pain, and reproductive organ complications.

It's important to also consider that reversing stress, or managing it better, can also help improve how our bodies are functioning in all these areas. As I've mentioned before, the two are linked bidirectionally, so they impact each other in both directions (positively and negatively).

Knowing all this, let's now consider some common chronic inflammatory conditions and their mental health symptoms. People who have lupus often struggle with mental disorientation and memory loss. Those who suffer with irritable bowel syndrome have common symptoms of anxiety. One of the major symptoms in fibromyalgia is depression. Chronic inflammation worsens negative mood states, and those mood states negatively impact the physical condition. These connected conditions become cyclical between the mind and the body. That's why when you work on *improving* either inflammation or mood, it will have a *positive* impact on the other. And this is why some medications that are used to treat inflammatory conditions also help alleviate mood. For example, drugs that treat rheumatoid arthritis, psoriasis, and asthma have had greater success in treating depression than some antidepressants, depending on the person being treated. A first-line defense against stress, therefore, would also focus on the reduction of inflammation in the body, which is why I stress it so much here. Because I don't want you to place a Band-Aid on your healing. I want you to be fully informed and globally heal your generational stress and strain.

Healing the Body, Holistically

A well-integrated trauma protocol will teach you how to help your body dissolve stress. In order to focus on healing the whole you rather than just treating one specific health condition, it will be essential for us to integrate holistic wellness practices into your daily routine. Whenever you move to heal with intention and intuition, a bit of your intergenerational trauma leaves your body. And it leaves room for your body to take in intergenerational health instead. Should you choose it, holistic wellness can be a new way of life.

Ancient cultures have been correcting the imbalances of the mind-body-spirit for generations. Humans have been using the earth's natural resources and energy to alleviate and treat illness for over sixty thousand years. There's a reason why healing practices have stuck around for millennia: because they work.

Holistic practices stimulate a healing response that offers serenity to your entire body. They include anything that falls under the umbrella of alternative medicine, homeopathy, or naturopathy, and include wisdom gathered from Ayurveda, Chinese medicine, African-derived healing, Indigenous wisdom, spiritualism, and a multitude of other schools of healing that have helped keep the human population alive for centuries. Holistic practitioners integrate a wide range of practices into their therapy depending on their training and the needs of the clients they serve. These practices can range from meditation to herb consumption, yoga to African dance movement therapy, teas to energy healing. They are honoring the body of wisdom that humanity has carried across the world.

One of my chosen techniques to integrate into my own life and into my work with clients is mindful tea making using botanical healing herbs. Botanicals are a special part of how I offer holistic-centered psychological education. Many people who are familiar with my work through social media know me for hosting what I call tea therapy sessions. I started filming therapy session–like videos while I made my favorite teas, providing some healing nuggets of wisdom while we were locked down during the COVID-19 pandemic. I used my signature catchphrase—*The tea is hot!*—to signify that the message I was delivering was going to be a tough but necessary point to digest about trauma, relationships, and mental health. And people appreciated it. What most people don't know about my teatime sessions is that they grew out of a deep, multigenerational love for tea and a family tradition of healing with tea.

After my grandmother passed, I started doing some healing work of my own, digging into my ancestry and gathering wisdom from my titi (my aunt); my great-uncle; my sister, Lady; my cousin Leezet; and my parents. That research is what first led me to tea. My mother makes tea every night. One night she offered me tea that smelled like lemongrass, my preferred scent for aromatherapy. As my mother made the tea, she explained to me how my grandmother would make the same tea back in Barahona. She started talking about my ancestral roots and the ways my family have relied on local tea blends as healing balms for many generations. My grandmother lived in a tiny little home in Barahona, in a community of Dominicans who have been deeply economically impoverished for generations. Her home was made of flimsy wood panels and had a tin roof, no floors (the ground was actual dirt), and no indoor plumbing. She had a makeshift kitchen, and in that kitchen, she brewed ancient wisdom. She steeped local herbs to help heal her children, including my mother, whenever they would come down with a sickness. Now, my mother was transferring that intergenerational wisdom to me, through my grandmother's lemongrass tea.

When I was younger, I always shrugged off my mother's belief in the restorative power of teas. Now I can't believe I ever took them for granted. When I smell lemongrass, I feel deeply grounded. Listening to my mother's story, I finally understood why. That scent was a source of healing for generations in my family. We can carry multigenerational scent memories that remind us of resilience and healing, much as I have with my grandmother's tea. After I first learned about these teas, I continued to dig. I discovered the many healing properties that were present in this particular tea blend—it had so many anti-inflammatory benefits. My mind was blown. I believe my grandmother would have wanted everyone to know about this tea, so they, too, could feel its healing power. So as a heartfelt intergenerational gift from my family to yours, I would like to offer you this recipe. I call it Mamá Tutúna's Lemongrass Healing Tea. And in case you need a little guidance on how it can help, I offer you some of the healing wisdom offered to me. You can find both this recipe and the information at the end of this book, in appendix A.

Breaking the Cycle: Stimulating the Intergenerational Ventral Vagus Nerve

Since your body is layered and ancestral, the work that you will be required to do to regulate it will also be layered. Vagal toning is a practice that helps go deep into your nervous system and stimulate your ventral vagus nerve—the nerve that has been known to be primarily responsible for nervous system rest and stress reduction. It's a practice that helps you enter into a calmer state. Stimulating the ventral vagus can produce an immediate effect upon your nervous system and can have a lasting effect on your overall emotional functioning. But how?

Vagus nerve stimulation (VNS) releases chemical signals called neuromodulators to your neurons to help increase the amount of "happy chemicals," like dopamine, serotonin, endorphins, and oxytocin, they produce. The VNS process sends signals to your neurons that you are safe, and as a result, these neuromodulators start to generate very specific and long-lasting changes in the brain. We call this neuroplasticity: when chemical shifts produce structural changes in certain brain regions. VNS has been successful in effectively helping the effects of some mild brain injuries and post-traumatic stress disorder. In short, it helps your body feel more at ease and can lessen the impact that trauma has had on your brain and nervous system, leaving greater opportunity for you to feel safe, widening your intergenerational window of tolerance (more on this in chapter 6, where we cover your intergenerational nervous system), and detoxifying the intergenerational stress in your body. So, in the spirit of using vagal nerve stimulation to offer you a tool for stress release, think back to a song that brings you into a loving, calm, easeful state. If the song is an oldie, like one that a loving family member or ancestor sang to you, it's an even better choice.

- Sit in a comfortable seat, if you are able, and lower your gaze to where it feels safe or fully close your eyes.
- If possible, place your right hand on your heart and your left hand on your belly.
- Take in a gentle breath, and start to hum the song.
- Be sure to monitor your breath, hum the tune very slowly, and pay close attention to how your body is taking in these sound vibrations.
- Imagine your hum deeply penetrating your nervous system and offering you healing, working its way through each one of your

neurons and creating new, healing-centered neural connections and cellular memory.

- Midway through the song, think of the people in your lineage whom you would like to see liberated from the burden of stress.
- Deepen your hum by humming a bit louder now, and as you deepen it, imagine your hum vibrating into their ventral vagal nerves.
- Keep them in mind as you hum the song to the very end.
- Imagine feeling calmer in your more regulated emotional state. Imagine that your family members do too. Imagine that your ancestors also feel this. Imagine how you are all collectively healing in this moment.
- Once you finish the song, feel free to catch another gentle breath to complete your practice.
- Send gratitude to the ancestors whom you have gathered into this practice with you by simply uttering the words "thank you."
- Give yourself a gentle squeeze.
- Open your eyes and sit for 30 more seconds.
- Observe what you feel. How's your soul in this moment?
- If it helps, grab your journal and take a moment to reflect on paper. I'm sure there's a lot to write.

What You've Learned So Far

In this chapter, you explored how stress is interpreted in the mind-body connection. You also learned how stress can be the culprit of many physical diseases and how holistic healing helps the body feel more settled. You then did an exercise that focused on the toning of your ventral vagal nerve. You learned a lot and did a lot, so congratulate yourself for getting through this bit, take a few deep breaths to continue to settle your body, and when you're ready, dive into your chapter's reflection questions, before heading into what intergenerational trauma truly is and how it lives in you.

REFLECTION QUESTIONS

What struck you most about how intergenerational trauma gets captured in the body?

How are you feeling about integrating holistic healing practices as a lifestyle or routine?

How was it for you to engage in the ventral vagal exercise offered in this chapter?

CHAPTER 4

Unhealed Trauma and You

Find freedom in the context you inherit.
—Revolutionary Stó:lō Indigenous author Lee Maracle

Now that you've gotten a good grasp on why you're reading this book—because you're a cycle breaker, because you have so much resilience that you carry within you, and because you deserve to heal the whole you—let's start understanding the greater depths of intergenerational trauma. When a physical body wound is left unhealed, it continues to cause pain and becomes vulnerable to infection. That infection and pain can spread to other parts of your body. Something similar happens with emotions. Negative emotions hurt us deeply when they are left unhealed. They have the power to contaminate every other part of our lives, making it feel, at times, almost unbearable to live. But unlike physical wounds, emotional wounds can reach beyond the person who is hurt and have the capacity to hurt others, like family members, significant others, friends, coworkers, and children. For this reason, unhealed emotional wounds can have devastating effects on entire families and entire communities.

Nola's Chronic Emptiness

People living with intergenerational trauma oftentimes experience chronic mental health symptoms. One of the most common conditions they have to cope with is depression. And that was certainly the case for Nola. Nola, my client who had idiopathic lung disease, had been struggling with something I dubbed "chronic emptiness." It was a chronic depression that had made it so that she couldn't find joy in her life, no matter how hard she tried. She couldn't even find joy in the two areas of life where she felt most accomplished: motherhood and her career. Nothing filled the void. Because depression does this. It creates deep sadness, emptiness, and loneliness. For Nola, her depression also manifested as ongoing irritability. She was always reacting negatively to those around her and would have frequent angry outbursts. That was her trauma response—or put differently, her emotional response to extreme distress.

Nola would find herself in frequent conflict with the people in her life, often picking arguments with those around her (her husband, her coworkers, the one friend she had managed to hold on to, and even her teenage daughter). Inescapable misery was all she knew, because growing up, it was all she saw. Her mother suffered the same emptiness, as had her grandmother. All of them were stuck in a cycle of misery.

As her doctor, I found it so hard to see how frequently Nola spiraled, especially at work. She was a social worker, and instead of helping heal her community through that work, she carried that same misery into her interactions with the people she was meant to assist. She talked down to them, was often irritable, and wouldn't help them with simple tasks that could keep them out of shelters. As they say, misery loves company, and Nola was one to spread her misery to everyone who came in contact with her. As in Nola's case, the hurt that one person experiences can become a harmful weapon that is discharged onto anyone nearby.

Many types of trauma responses exist, and their manifestations can vary drastically from person to person. However, trauma responses are unified in that they are caused by suffering and create new suffering. They create suffering for others, as was the case with Nola, and create suffering for yourself, like in the examples of self-harm, self-destruction, or binge drinking.

How do you know if what you are experiencing is a trauma response? For starters, a part of you intuitively knows that your response is coming from a place of overwhelming stress. This stress can be acute (meaning that the traumatic experience caused a sudden, high level of emotional strain and perhaps even threatened your life, like a natural disaster, a theft at gunpoint, or a serious accident), or it can be chronic (meaning that the stressor happened over a long period of time, like childhood abuse, oppression, or toxic family dynamics).

But a trauma response isn't the original, traumatic event itself. It's how you emotionally processed the event. It's how your mind coped with the harmful circumstance in order to keep you alive and safe. So, when you're experiencing a trauma response, in reality what you're experiencing are mental adaptations that are designed to keep you sane and keep your mind and heart intact through an overwhelming event. The problem arises when those symptoms carry on once you're no longer threatened but you still feel the need to incessantly protect yourself.

Trauma itself, according to present-day clinical definitions of trauma, can fall into multiple categories, including post-traumatic stress, childhood trauma, complex trauma, race-based trauma, and, now, intergenerational trauma. Some of these representations of trauma have not yet made it into the diagnostic manual that clinicians use across the world. But you don't need a scientific manual to tell you that your experience is genuine, or that your lived experience is one that's been impacted by emotional hurt. You feel the harm in your *mind* through your emotions and thoughts, in your *body* through physical sensations and triggers, and through your *spirit* in your broken relationships, your lack of feeling grounded, and your sense that you're always in survival mode. You feel it in your *soul*. I know this is a lot to take in. You may be feeling the weight of all this as you read. But don't worry, I've got you, and we will be learning a lot of practices that can help.

How Do You Know You Are Dealing with Intergenerational Trauma?

So where do you even begin? Well, you may have guessed this already, but it starts with identifying what brought you to pick up this book in the first place. In my own experience, my first understanding of how I was carrying intergenerational wounds came when I recognized my inability to let go of small material things as a symptom of trauma. For you, the first time that you knew that you had been experiencing intergenerational trauma may have been when you had to create a healthy distance with a family member. Perhaps it was when you first noticed that you had your emotions invalidated by your family members your whole life. Or maybe it was when you realized that you reacted to stress and emotional hurt in the very same ways that your parents did. Or maybe it was when:

- You went to therapy and realized that you've seen your unhealthy adult relationship patterns reflected in your childhood home.
- You realized that a large part of your emotional suffering comes from not receiving enough love from your caretakers, and that they, too, suffered the same fate.
- You noticed that you were repeating the same toxic relationship cycles that you saw your parents cycling through.
- You realized that your family was keeping deep secrets that have plagued them—and you—emotionally.

- You started seeing that the relationship dynamics in your family are actually toxic and harmful, rather than seeing them as the norm.
- You realized that you have a history of people-pleasing in order to feel accepted and loved and that this history started in your family long before you were conceived.
- You noticed that your relationships have had codependent patterns, which you've always assumed were standard in relationships.
- You realized that it was considered normal for your family to gaslight each other.
- You realized that despite your consciousness around unhealthy relationships, you continued to behave in ways that have been harmful, even to your own children.
- You wondered why abusive relationships felt like home and why others in your family have felt the same.
- You realized that you tend to zone out whenever you don't feel safe around people and recall past generations also zoning out when life felt too stressful.
- You realized that you were subconsciously resorting to addiction to numb your pain in the same ways that people in your family have.
- The loss of a family member brought up some emotions that you thought were buried.
- You heard the story of an ancestor's life and realized how similar their suffering has been to your own.
- You noticed how hard it was for you to trust both yourself and others, in the very same ways it was for your parents to trust.
- You realized that you found it hard to accept love from others, because genuine love wasn't shown to you, and now as an adult, expressions of love have made you feel uncomfortable.
- You realized that it was hard for you to tell people that you loved them, because it was never modeled for you.

- You had your own children and started worrying about the possibility that you might pass down the same emotional stressors you inherited from your parents.
- You noticed yourself repeating the same harmful language and punishment to your children.
- You realized that belonging to a marginalized group has been a source of suffering for your family well before you were born.
- You realized that you and your lineage had been victimized by institutions for generations.
- You started realizing that there were undiagnosed and untreated mental health challenges and traumas in your family.
- You couldn't gather any medical explanation for your symptoms.
- You realized that your family was also operating from a hurt place, and as hurtful as it has been to acknowledge, you had to sit with the fact that this was the best they could do.
- You realized you deserved a better past and desired a better future.

One or more of these may sound exactly like the moment(s) that drove you to know that you'd been struggling with the anxiety, depression, sadness, shame, loneliness, and trauma of people who came before you. Or your story may be different still. There are many more moments of realization that don't fit into this list but are factual and painful experiences that you've had to endure and that signal intergenerational trauma. Whatever your story is, hold it close to your heart. It is yours and it is valid. Regardless of which moments made you realize that you had layers of trauma in your family life, you are here, with an elevated consciousness of the fact that intergenerational wounds have afflicted your family and that they flow through you. And I know that it can be traumatizing in itself to come to terms with the idea that trauma is a part of your lineage. We will slowly draft your intergenerational narrative through the mapping of your history in an Intergenerational Trauma Healing Assessment and the creation of your Intergenerational Trauma Tree in this and the following chapter. We will also talk about how to manage the emotions that come up when you start digging through the layers, so you'll be prepared each step of the way. For now, know that as you read along, right here and right now, you have in you the power and opportunity to break the cycle of pain. And as hard as it is to be the one to have to do this work, you should also be proud to pivot the destiny of your entire lineage. That's no easy feat, but here you are, doing it nevertheless.

Intergenerational Strain: What Our Ancestors Felt

All our lived experiences taken together—from distant ancestors, to living ancestors, to you—can culminate in a layering of *intergenerational strain*. I like to call it strain because that's exactly what it does. It overtaxes you. It's a burden that you carry, and even if you carry it with honor, it still feels strenuous and it makes life that much more difficult to bear. Intergenerational strain lives within you, and it is a mental, physical, spiritual, and cultural transmission of trauma. It is the multigenerational distress that accumulates, becomes engrained in your soul, and determines the way you engage with life's woes *and* joys.

Long before inherited trauma was conceptualized in our various fields of modern medicine, humans showed signs of understanding this phenomenon from the perspective of energetic, soul-based transmissions. In some Afro-Indigenous cultures, a person who experiences a psychological crisis is seen as someone who is in deep connection to their spiritual inner world. They are believed to be carrying a spiritual gift, lost somewhere in their lineage, that needs to be recovered by the community. Similarly, among Native Americans, people experiencing stress are thought to be carrying sorrows from up to seven generations of their lineage. If they don't achieve resolution in their generation, that stress is said to affect up to seven generations into the future.

If we reflect on descendance dating seven generations back, we are looking at 128 fifth great-grandparents, who bore 64 of their children, who bore 32 of their children, who bore 16 of their children, who bore 8 of their children, who bore your 4 grandparents, who bore your 2 parents, who, finally, bore *you*. Taken together, and counting only seven generations back, you carry at least 255 direct histories in you, including your own. This awakening to how many potential soul wounds you carry within you is an important step in healing.

We are getting ready to dive into your lineage in more detail. As we do, take this advice: Treat your lineage reflections as a data collection practice. Collect this data and analyze it as if you were in a research lab, looking for answers, patterns, and solutions. In part, this book is a journey of data collection, knowledge attainment, and ancestral analysis. In these pages you will be learning and unlearning, finding the best solutions to set you on the best path forward, and developing within you intergenerational abundance. So, let's recap for a moment:

- Intergenerational strain refers to the mind, body, spirit, and cultural transmission of trauma.
- Yes, your genes play a role that makes this a unique type of trauma. We'll cover this concept in detail in the next chapter, when we learn about epigenetics.
- Yes, this is in large part linked to what your parents and ancestors went through.
- Yes, there's a lot of history living in you right now.
- Yes, you do have to do some heavy lifting to feel lighter.
- Yes, that heavy lifting will require you looking at layers of trauma strain.
- No, trauma doesn't determine your whole life, but it can make life heavier to carry.
- Yes, in the pages to come, you will continue to learn ways to shed some of that weight.

Breaking the Cycle: The Intergenerational Trauma Healing Assessment

After identifying that you are suffering from intergenerational trauma, the next step toward breaking the cycle is gathering information about what has contributed to the cycle in the first place. To that end, I have created an assessment that addresses the multiple areas of intergenerational trauma. I call it the Intergenerational Trauma Healing Assessment. This assessment offers a starting point for information gathering about how this layered trauma has shown up in your life. It can be used as both a tool for your healing and as a resource for healers who are helping clients with intergenerational pain. The questions in this assessment offer an opportunity for a baseline reflection on your own intergenerational trauma experiences. The exploration that you devote to each of these questions can be as in-depth as you feel is necessary.

Now, it's important to note that the setup for the assessment will be just as important as the assessment itself. You will figure out what type of preparation and setting works best for you, but here are some ideas to get you started:

- Find a healing space that embodies groundedness, tranquility, and safety. This place can be in your home, or maybe it's in an outdoor space. I've created several of these spaces in my home. Some are indoors and some out. Feel free to designate a number of spaces to your healing. The key here is that when you combine groundedness, tranquility, and safety, you've got a healthy physical setup for your depth work. It can be useful to have an item in that space that helps you feel grounded, like a comfort blanket or an item that someone has gifted you that makes you feel appreciated and seen. Any item works, so long as it contributes to the safe and tranquil ambiance we are aiming for. You can additionally set the scene with candles and gentle aromatic oils that you can either smell or massage into your hands when you need extra grounding. An essential element of safety is privacy, so choose spaces that grant you an opportunity to establish privacy to do this depth work.

- Locate an item that holds a story or energy in your home. This can be a family heirloom or it can be your sage, palo santo, yerba santa, crystals, holy water, or other energy-producing objects that hold value in your life. You might wish to invite these items into your space to offer a more profound energetic experience to your assessment practice.

- Once you've established where you'd like to be, and what items you'd like to be surrounded by, it is imperative that you find a moment to ground yourself and bring yourself as close as possible to safely being in your body and in your mind in the present moment. This can be a moment to dive into the accompanying sound bath meditation for this section. For some additional ideas, look in appendix B for a list of Intergenerational Trauma Healing Grounding Techniques.

- Finally, you will need courage. This is vulnerable work. Vulnerable work is brave work. All of it produces fear, and all of it requires that you dip into that core generational resilience that you have within you.

Remember to pace yourself. This assessment is yours and it is to be done on your own time and at a pace that feels aligned. Don't force the journey. Instead, flow. Begin the Intergenerational Trauma Healing Assessment on the following page by answering each question. Take as long as you need to answer each question thoroughly. And as much as you're able, try not to skip any questions, even when your answers are short and especially when your answers are difficult to face. Remember to breathe and that you've got the generational strength you need to proceed.

INTERGENERATIONAL TRAUMA HEALING ASSESSMENT
Checking In

- How are you feeling about starting this assessment?
- Run a body scan: check in with your body, and notice any sensations. What is your body remembering?
- Write down how you feel about the practice and your body's memories or sensations that have come up as you think about this assessment.
- Remember to anchor yourself with a grounding technique or this section's sound bath meditation at all points in the assessment, but especially before you get started.

Mapping Your Origins

Answer the below questions with a few sentences to describe how these experiences have shown up in your own family:

- In what way has anyone in your family used the word *trauma* to describe experiences they have had? This includes you, by the way.
- What experiences were referenced to regarding trauma?
- Have there been incidents of psychological, physical, or sexual abuse within your family? If so, which ones? Be as descriptive as you can be while being mindful of your internal experience of writing these down. Reflections on abuse can feel triggering, so note how you're emotionally metabolizing these reflections and offer yourself pauses and recalibration with grounding techniques as needed.
- Have there been longstanding separations (e.g., due to divorce, immigration, loss of a home, and others)? If so, what happened?
- Have there been experiences of addiction in your family? If so, write down anything that feels relevant to those experiences.

- Have there been adverse medical experiences in your lineage? If so, what have these been?
- Have there been people in your family who have experienced a sudden or unexpected death? If so, what happened? And how did people process that loss?
- Have there been experiences of cultural violence in your family (e.g., racism, poverty, religious discrimination, land abduction, occupation, identity bias, cultural depravation, wars, and others)? If so, what have these been? Add as much context as you need.
- In what ways has there been an air of silence around family issues?
- In what ways have trauma responses been normalized in your family? How have they been normalized in your community?
- Have there been other experiences that have felt vastly overwhelming that are unique to your family of origin or communities? Detail these as needed and remember to add details pertaining to each generation that you have information about.

Your Inner Knowing
- When did you first realize that you had inherited intergenerational trauma?
- What happened during that moment of realization?
- Where in your body have you felt the wounds of generational pain?
- What bodily sensations come up for you now as you reflect?
- What emotions come up as you think about having an inheritance of trauma?
- How did you feel in relation to your family members when you came to this realization?
- How did you feel in relation to yourself when you figured out that you had been suffering from intergenerational trauma?

Qualifying the Impact

- How has intergenerational trauma contributed to your feeling either connected or disconnected from others?
- Where has it caused a disruption or unease in your family life?
- In which ways has it caused a disruption in your life (e.g., in your relationships, career, etc.)?
- In what ways have you inherited intergenerational strength and resilience?
- What generational wisdom have you gathered from people in your family and community?
- In what ways has that wisdom helped you survive hard moments?
- In what ways is that generational strength helping you navigate the healing presented in this book?

You and the Work

- What aspects of your generational inheritance are you intentionally holding on to?
- What aspects of your generational inheritance are you ready to let go of?
- When you imagine a version of yourself that is operating from a place of healing, what comes to mind?
- When you see yourself well into this journey, what would make your soul feel at ease?
- What are three grounding techniques that you are willing to commit to daily as you do this depth work beyond this assessment? (See appendix B for a list of grounding techniques to try.)

Checking Out

- How are you feeling after going through this assessment? What emotions are still present? (Mind)
- Check in with yourself through a body scan and notice any sensations. Where is your body remembering? (Body)

- How connected or distanced are you feeling toward your lineage and yourself? (Spirit)

As you end the assessment, remember to anchor yourself with your chosen grounding technique or this section's sound bath meditation. You've done something major and hard. Take however long you need to let everything sink in. And treat yourself to some moments of calm to help settle any emotions that linger. When you're ready, let's conclude this exercise and seal it with a final round of deep breaths. Breathe in deeply and out fully until your body feels safe and well.

What You've Learned So Far

In this chapter, you learned to identify intergenerational trauma and how you can spot it in your own lineage. We rounded out the chapter by helping you work back into your own history through the Intergenerational Trauma Healing Assessment to start digging into the ways in which intergenerational trauma and resilience have shown up in your life and the impact they have had. Are you ready to keep going? I hope so, and I especially hope you feel grounded and filled with the courage you'll require for the work ahead. Take a quick dive into your reflection questions, and let's get into the genetics of it all.

REFLECTION QUESTIONS

What was your aha moment when you knew you had a history of intergenerational trauma?

How did you feel when completing the Intergenerational Trauma Healing Assessment?

What lessons did you take in about how you relate to your own intergenerational trauma after completing the assessment?

CHAPTER 5

A Genetic Inheritance

Hijos de tigres nacen con rayas.
(Children of tigers are born with their stripes.)
—Latine expression, told by my mother, Margarita

Intergenerational trauma is a force that flows from one generation of a family to the next. The emotions that don't get resolved or attended to in one generation risk being passed down, again and again. Your family's trauma has become both a biological and a social inheritance that eventually made its way to you. It's a legacy that perpetuates because most people don't know how to identify it, claim it, or do the work to resolve it. People who have a history of intergenerational trauma have a parent (or two), grandparents, great-grandparents, and more distant ancestors who have experienced their own traumas. Those living with unresolved intergenerational trauma are often not fully aware of its symptoms or dangers, so they have little opportunity, and even fewer resources, to work through it. This might be because they haven't been informed about what intergenerational trauma is, since it's one of the newer areas of study in mental health, but also because these traumas have been so widely normalized across communities that

69

they've become almost invisible. And what isn't seen is difficult to work through. In some cases, it's impossible. Most often, this leads to inter-generational trauma unwittingly being passed on, from one person to the next.

There are levels to consider here. There are what we call *big-T trau-mas* (traumas that are extreme and pervasive and threaten your safety or person) and *little-*t *traumas*, or subtle traumas (situations that are common, day-to-day occurrences that cause emotional injury but don't create a threat to your safety).

The big-*T* and little-*t* traumas of your ancestors, matched with the ways in which they responded to these experiences, were then transmitted to you, first at the genetic level as you were forming into life in the womb, and later, in the ways that you experienced the world, through ongoing stressors and through the modeling of how to cope through those very issues. This is not an exhaustive list of big-*T* and little-*t* traumas, but take a look to see if any of these sound familiar.

Big-*T* Traumas Can Be

- Having been abandoned by caretakers
- Living with parents who don't attend to your needs (physical, emotional, or spiritual)
- Not having your basic needs cared for (e.g., clean clothes, proper nutrition, hygiene), even if this was not an intentional act but a byproduct of the economic injustice your caregivers suffered
- Your parents getting a divorce, especially if the divorce included heavy emotional and logistical turmoil
- Having loved ones who were addicted to substances or suffered other addictions
- Having your body boundaries violated, such as through molestation and sexual violence

- Experiencing extreme forms of punishment
- Having a parent experience incarceration
- Experiencing identity-based injustice or persecution
- Being forced to assimilate to a new culture or language
- Being displaced from your home
- Living in poverty
- Living in a war-stricken or occupied land
- Experiencing or witnessing violence or bodily harm
- Being bullied
- Suffering from, or having someone close to you suffer from, a debilitating illness
- Having a medical experience go wrong
- Experiencing a serious accident
- Experiencing a natural disaster or pandemic
- Witnessing a death
- And having any other experience that threatened your sense of safety, identity, or well-being

Little-*t* Traumas Can Be

- Having to relocate to a new town or land
- Losing a treasured pet
- Experiencing ongoing conflict with someone
- Disclosing something vulnerable and being invalidated as a result
- Being scapegoated, that is, being the target of someone else's frustrations and anger
- Losing a treasured item
- Working with a difficult supervisor or colleague
- Going through a bad breakup
- Having a temporary financial emergency
- Experiencing sudden changes in your family
- Losing a part of your support system

- Experiencing a non-life-threatening injury
- Not getting a job you wanted
- Being rejected by a friend or love interest
- Going through a legal battle
- Having to hide who you are
- Being in a toxic relationship (but one that did not threaten your sense of safety)
- And experiencing just about anything else that could be perceived as highly stressful but does not cause a high-level safety threat

No matter the level of trauma or the impact it produced, the way that a trauma is internalized can be very individual and personal, which means that any trauma has the capacity to create the experience of generational traumatization. Don't underestimate the power of little-*t* traumas when compounded over time. All traumatic experiences, big *and* little, have the capacity to make us feel emotionally overburdened. With enough nurturing, big-*T* traumas can go away, and with an unhealthy-enough emotional environment, little-*t* traumas can have a massive, intergenerational impact. That is to say, the level of the traumatic experience itself isn't the only thing that can keep trauma going. Our social environments also play a large part in how these big-*T* and little-*t* traumas get processed.

It Starts with a Strong Environment

Stressful social environments or, as some cognitive behavioral therapists call them, *strong environments*, can leave an imprint on your epigenome—your gene expressions—and cause myriad potentially devastating consequences for you and your descendants. A strong environment is one where stress is persistently high, like a home with a bad-tempered parent, or a neighborhood where your safety was constantly threatened, or a school where you lived in a state of terror due to bullies or violence. When that stress persists for months or even years, you register the stress caused by your strong environment in your very cells.

Much of our initial understanding of genetic transmissions of trauma came from studies involving the descendants of Holocaust survivors. This extreme environment, in which terror and genocide persisted in concentration camps that were defined by brutal violence, endless death, violations of safety, and constant terror, left deep emotional scars on the survivors. What scientists found to be remarkable was that the remnants of that trauma were also apparent through generations of their descendants.

And so, to understand those remnants, the most notable studies in my field focus not on the Holocaust survivors themselves but rather on the children of survivors and the intergenerational transmission of trauma responses that they carried. These studies are notable because they showed that adult children of Holocaust survivors had a unique genetic marker: their cortisol levels were below the levels of Jewish people who had not been born to Holocaust survivors, and low cortisol levels can be indicative of the presence of PTSD. There was a distinct difference in the cortisol levels of descendants from sufferers of persistent horror and those who did not carry that legacy. And studies continue to show the adverse effects of these big-T traumas on groups of targeted communities, including people of the African diaspora, due to the centuries of racial terror, caste systems, and oppression that continue to cause multigenerational harm to people of African descendance. Similar work has focused on the risk of mental illness among Native Americans, given that multiple generations have suffered genocide, terror, and displacement at the hands of European colonizers. And other studies have also begun to focus on the generational experiences of Aboriginal people, Asian communities, South Asian communities,

Middle Eastern communities, and other populations who have amassed collective traumas and for whom trauma has been passed down for centuries.

How Trauma Gets Stuck

We all have a hardwired neurological system to help us deal with stress, and your body responds automatically to help you resolve it and move on from it. When you're presented with a stressor, you enter a state of alarm. Your nervous system is activated by the release of stress hormones, namely cortisol and adrenaline. At this stage, physically, your pupils dilate, your heart rate increases, your breath shortens, your senses heighten, and you may even start to tremble. Your body is preparing to fend off the threat. Typically, once the stressor is dealt with or disappears and your nervous system no longer perceives a threat to your safety, your body prepares to rest after being so energized. Those stress hormones start to flush out of your system as you calm down and achieve emotional balance. For example, a milder way in which this might happen is presented in the following scenario. You have to go to a doctor's appointment and need to make sure you have your referral slip to receive the service. However, you can't find the slip. You are at risk of being late and missing your appointment, so your stress hormones elevate. But fortunately you find the slip, just in time to make it to your appointment, at which time your nervous system no longer feels alarmed. So it naturally relaxes. The threat of missing your appointment is gone. You are back in balance. That's a way in which a daily occurrence can bring your nervous system to a heightened state and then into balance once it no longer needs to be on alert.

But what if the stressor does not go away? What if the stress is entirely too powerful to dissipate on its own? Or what if you are exposed to the same stressful event over and over again? If the stress lingers for an extended time, say, days or weeks, then you may start to develop certain signs of ongoing emotional unrest. This may eventually instigate persistent emotional symptoms like sadness, poor concentration, and irritability, and physical complications like bowel problems, headaches, and sleeplessness. If you can't resolve these symptoms in a reasonable amount of time and your mind and body are not allowed to rest, you will be stressed beyond your capacity to cope and your body's resources will be exhausted. If this level of stress exists in a body for years on end, that's when a person becomes susceptible to chronic illness, disease, and even death. More often than not, when this chronic stress is left unaddressed, it becomes an emotional inheritance.

In recent decades, our understanding of the nervous system and how it's implicated in trauma responses has surged forward. Traumatic symptoms have been identified as being incomplete physical responses detained in the body. The body captures energy connected to each situation we are engaged in. And when a life-threatening or a chronically stressful event happens, it becomes energy in the body that seeks to be discharged. If it's held in the body for too long, that energy can develop into a symptom of trauma, which is very often difficult to expel.

The body holds a memory of the stressful event, which makes it harder for the body to process and release that energy the next time a stressor is encountered. That bodily energy becomes frozen. Held in the body for too long, the cumulative energy will eventually be converted into the undercurrent of intergenerational trauma, because our nervous system is set up to move through stress and discharge it quickly, not hold on to it. If you're not able to emancipate that stress-based energy from your body successfully, then it becomes stuck, debilitating, and in time, intergenerational.

Picture this: You're riding in an elevator and you hear a big thump. You try to open the door and realize you're stuck. The call button doesn't work. An hour goes by, then two, and still, no one has heard your screams for help. Tension is building up inside you. With every passing moment, more energy accumulates. Your heart is beating continuously at a mile a minute, your breath is constricting, your body begins to tremble, and you become dizzy. Your thoughts are telling you that you'll never be found. You're now fearing death. And so, your entire body is now in an energetic upsurge, trying to keep you alive.

When help finally arrives, your body is still responding to the fear you felt in the elevator. The stressor might be gone, but the stress in your body remains. You don't immediately enter the rest state. Release comes when you actively help your nervous system relax, either through deep breaths or other relaxation practices. If you never get a chance to actively calm down, you risk not recovering a sense of safety in your body. Without initiating that calming process, either naturally or intentionally, your body can become stuck in the feeling of surviving a threat. This stuck energy then can become a trauma symptom. Months later, the fear and the bodily responses that accompanied that stressor become chronic. Years later, your body resorts to fear as the norm, and your cells register that your body is chronically in trauma.

Several scientific areas of study are working to help us weave together the pieces of this massive web we call intergenerational trauma. To give you a sense of the widespread importance of intergenerational trauma, consider that critical information regarding generational transmissions can be found in fields focused on the structure and function of our cells (cellular biology); the contents of the mind (psychology); the biological process of emotions (psychiatry); the brain structure (neurology); the ways the nervous system and brain influence the mind (neuropsychology); prenatal development of sex cells, embryos, and fetuses (embryology); the connection between the mind, body, and relationships (interpersonal neurobiology); the relationship between immunity, the endocrine system, and nervous system (psychoneuroimmunology); the ways early life adversity leads to adult impairment (developmental science); and, most notably, how our social environments affect our gene expressions (epigenetics).

Each of these fields of scientific inquiry has played a key part in revealing the importance of generational histories. Each has played a role in revealing the multitude of ways in which traumatic experiences are held in the mind, body, and spirit, which then impact a vast number of people. Each field has helped us understand a key aspect of how traumatic stress impacts us at the microscopic, cellular level, and interestingly, how this transmission might have begun long before we were born.

Three Bodies in One

Researchers and scientists are finding that bodies tell stories through the remnants of stress left in their cells. And it begins at, well, the beginning. The initial mechanism of trauma transmission is through sex cells (through both the egg and sperm) at conception. Studies conducted specifically on sperm have found that stress-related gene expressions are reflected in those cells. Sperm cells multiply throughout a person's life span, replicating genetic messages that include the cellular memory of trauma. The other type of sex cell, the ovum, or egg cell— although it doesn't replicate the way that sperm cells do—carries similar genetic messages.

Fetuses develop their precursor sex cells in utero. That means you originated as a precursor egg and sperm cell in your parents' reproductive organs while *they* were still developing as embryos inside your grandmothers' uteruses. It's a beautiful transgenerational moment where you, your parents, and your grandmothers were all one. You were coexisting within each other on both your maternal and paternal sides; three generations in one body, sharing the same stories, sounds, vibrations, breaths, and love, but simultaneously, the same stressors. You were a part of two separate intergenerational bodies, which means that you shared these intergenerational womb experiences with your mother and maternal grandmother, but also with your father and paternal grandmother. Whatever thoughts and emotions were driving the lived experiences of both your grandmothers were pushing hormones into their bloodstream, which filtered to your parents, and to you. In these moments, the cells that you would later develop into were internalizing whatever was going on in your grandmothers' lives via those hormones. If they were stressed, then their stress hormones alerted all the cells in their pregnant bodies (including you!) to the fact that something didn't feel safe. The sex cells that were existing in these intergenerational wombs were susceptible to the stress they felt. The precursor cells that would eventually become you were taking emotional input from both of your grandmothers' social environments, and if they sensed stress was chronically present in their bodies, then it's likely that your genes were undergoing an epigenetic regulation, where cells register how they should respond to stimuli or stressors. Over time, any overstimulation or chronic stimulation to stress that was a part of that formation could have had an impact on your cognitive development, emotions, and nervous system—before your parents were even born.

It's Within Your Cells

When we're conceived, we inherit not just characteristics like eye color, hair, and height, but also personality characteristics and even how we cope with life's stressors. In fact, only 2 percent of genetic markers contribute to our external characteristics. All others are related to traits we can't see. In the 1980s, we learned that genes have the capacity to turn themselves on or off based on the signals they get from our social environment. These genes control not just how we look physically but also our emotions and behaviors. From this understanding of cell behavior, scientists and clinicians started to develop a window of knowledge into how an ancestor's cellular memory could alter the genetic expressions of their descendants. This was something that I saw come up very explicitly in my work with my longtime client Brooklyn.

Brooklyn was born a cycle breaker. She was inquisitive, so curious about everything. So it made sense that she would apply that curiosity to her family history. Brooklyn came from a home where chaos was the norm. "Everyone has something," she would say to me, in reference to her family's mental health histories. But she didn't see this as a fate she should resign herself to. "I won't let it define me," she would often say. And I believed her. I saw her will to break cycles, and I wanted to help.

When I started working with Brooklyn, she was in the third year of her undergraduate studies at a college in New York City. She is a native New Yorker, and at the time, she lived with her family and worked a part-time job while attending school. She had a revolutionary spirit with a level of inquisition that I believe was both her gift and her Achilles' heel. Her curiosity about her own emotional situation sometimes sent her down deep rabbit holes, which would eventually lead her to what we came to call her "deep grief." In this deep grief, Brooklyn would fear the worst (mind), experience chronic throbbing headaches (body), and feel completely disconnected from herself and everyone around her (spirit). In other words, she felt it in her soul. Because of the chaos of her family and home, Brooklyn lived in chronic stress. She was generally anxious, worrying about everything and everyone. She didn't have one stressor, but many. Brooklyn was disturbed when she noticed that as soon as things felt too good to be true, like when she received the excellent grades that she deserved, or when she felt more deeply connected to her romantic partner, she would go down the rabbit hole, digging deeper each time, until she found herself sabotaging the opportunity or the relationship and returning to her place of fear and darkness. Both Brooklyn and I were curious about what her deep grief could tell us about her family's past and the reasons why it felt so familiar and strangely comforting for her to go there.

What we learned is that this deep grief was more familiar to her and felt more like home than when she was surrounded by positivity and hope. She subconsciously sought it out when things felt too good. She told me, "Every cell in my body feels right when I go into that deep sorrow." And when I heard that, my eyes widened. Something major had clicked into place.

I went down my own rabbit hole to understand the scientific and psychological implications of that sentiment. I wanted to discover *how* her body was impacted by that impulse. It turns out, she wasn't too far off in saying that *every cell* felt her pain. When in trauma, certain cells actually do get activated, especially if they have been programmed to overreact to stress through generations of experiences. I was certain that there was a deep, ancestral, painful energy flowing through Brooklyn's whole body. And I was committed to helping her understand this for herself. I will highlight what Brooklyn's journey looked like in the chapters to come, but for now, let's dive deeper into how our bodies become wired to trauma at the cellular level.

Wired Together

We are biologically connected to the stress of our families in so many ways. One of the most powerful is through the nerve cells in our bodies called neurons. Neurons are a fundamental component of our nervous system, and they're responsible for taking in sensory information from the outside world. The messages neurons receive from the world are then sent to our bodies through electrical signals that get transferred as information to our brains. Every sensory experience you have—every sound, every touch, every smell, every taste, and every sight—is nothing more than an electrical charge that sends a message back from your body to your brain.

Now, if a neuron is reflective of how you experience the world through these electrical signals, then a mirror neuron is a neuron that fires an electrical charge when you are experiencing someone else's world. Let's say you're watching someone enter a dark attic on TV. If you feel afraid, it's not because you are in danger; it's because you suspect the person on the television might be in danger as they enter this dark, scary room. That fear is caused by your mirror neurons at work. You empathetically experience the emotions you believe others to be experiencing. When scientists began to study this feeling, they were able to see that the prefrontal areas of your brain that fire certain neurons when, for example, you enter a dark attic are connected to the neurons that fire when you watch someone else enter a dark attic.

Over time, after repeatedly taking in someone else's experience as your own, your mirror neurons have a greater chance of overfiring and start forming a habitual response to others' emotions. Overactive mirror neurons are especially prevalent in families with intense emotional exchanges and high levels of emotional reactivity. Mirror neurons help you create a sense of empathy, but if overused, they might make it hard to separate your emotional responses from someone else's.

In Brooklyn's home, everyone's emotional experiences were wired together. They mirrored each other's hurt with so much unconscious empathy that a single family member's dilemma could bring the whole family into a nervous system overdrive. This is something I call the *intergenerational nervous system*. I'll explain this more in the upcoming chapter, but just know that for Brooklyn and her family, it meant that when one person felt sorrow, another felt empathy for that sorrow, then another, then another, until everyone in her house was sad, or in deep grief. When one person felt anger, they all felt angry too. And so on. They shared a single emotional experience, triggered collectively. This is not uncommon in families where emotional chaos is the norm. These families collectively absorb the emotions felt by one individual, because they are all functioning under one collective mirror neuron experience.

I remember the instance when Brooklyn and I first discussed this phenomenon. She felt a sense of hopelessness at seeing how many layers of preprogramming she had been operating under for so many years. She was equally upset at finally comprehending the ways her family members had to suffer an emotional debt that didn't belong to them.

She was confronted with the reality that, in that very moment, while we sat in silence giving space to her tears, she couldn't immediately change these ingrained responses in her family or in herself. First, we had to sit with her layered frustration for her own pain and for the pain her family had suffered for generations. We had to sit with the fact that she had lived through critical periods in her life this way and that we couldn't turn back the clock to undo how her nervous system had been shaped by these intergenerational forces. The only thing we could do in that very moment was look forward. We didn't have the power to rewrite the past, but we could work our way through the discomfort and pain while we mapped out a way to help her restructure her own nervous system. Our goal was to help Brooklyn find some liberation.

Rather than being defeated, Brooklyn would leave my office that day with an elevated consciousness about how her family's stress responses were wired together. Ultimately, she felt that a weight had been lifted from her shoulders from finally knowing that she and her family were chronically triggered. Although it was hard information to sit with and although it did give her a sense of sadness, she also experienced relief. She looked at her own body with awe for how it had been syncing with the bodies of her family. And she felt a deep sense of agency over herself after this moment. She now understood something that could set her free from the contagion effect of stress that ran through her family's home. And that, to Brooklyn, was pure gold.

You will also have moments that feel insightful and empowering. Gaining a deeper knowledge about your own family's preprogramming will come with some grief, but it will also come with relief, as it did for Brooklyn. The work will ultimately be worth it.

That's a Trauma Response!

Trauma response is a term that seems to be taking over the world these days. A trauma response, to put it plainly, is a chronic reaction to a stressor. Trauma responses are how you learned to keep yourself safe. And they can be helpful (adaptive) or unhelpful (maladaptive). Some trauma responses can be passed down genetically or through behavior. Here is a milder example to help illustrate. Let's say your grandparent was badly burned on a stove when they were young, and so they held a lifelong fear of being burned by stoves. When you were a kid, they yelled "Watch out!" every time you got near one. Now, as an adult, that fear of hot stoves that was modeled by your grandparent has turned into your own fear of getting near a stove. The fear that you could get burned became so profound, in fact, that you've never learned to cook to avoid a burn. That's an inherited trauma response. It's a response that's driven by fear resulting from a traumatic experience of your ancestor. This fear belonged to someone else—your grandparent—was modeled for you, and subsequently instilled in you. Now you carry that trauma response too.

There are as many variations of trauma responses as there are people. As you start reflecting on which of your own behaviors might be trauma responses, remember that the purpose here isn't to shed light on these responses in order to produce shame in you. Rather, the purpose is to draw conscious attention to these behaviors with curiosity. In the best case, this will allow you to notice how you've operated from survival mode and why. Reflecting on which of your behaviors might be trauma responses is an exercise intended to help you draw out your own ancestral trauma patterns that are no longer helpful responses or adaptive ones. It's true, these trauma responses may have helped you, your family, and your community adapt and survive for generations. You may even see them as a familiar companion that you subconsciously don't want to let go of, like Brooklyn's "deep grief." And yet, recognizing these behaviors is the first step in helping you feel motivated to replace them with better ones. When you build your intergenerational trauma toolbox with the practices I propose throughout this book, you will have a wider range of ways to approach your healing. This will allow you to live a more fulfilled life and redefine your intergenerational legacy.

Before we can get to the goal of establishing your legacy, we must shed light on these trauma responses so you can begin to replace them with healthier behaviors. Let's start here: In your journal, list any trauma responses that you or your family carry. Keep them handy, because we will need them in the next section, when we start adding layers to this exercise. To help you begin, here are a few common examples of what trauma responses might look like:

- Avoiding confrontations at all costs
- Having a short fuse when stressed
- Shutting down at the slightest hint of stress
- Not talking about or expressing authentic emotions
- Not being able to show vulnerability in relationships
- Behaving in a self-destructive way that puts your well-being at risk
- Staying silent and perpetually not taking action
- Feeling chronically empty
- Having chronic pessimism and a negative outlook on life
- Experiencing long bouts of sadness
- Constantly operating from a place of fear
- Feeling jumpy and getting startled easily at sudden noises
- Being unable to concentrate
- Having upsetting dreams
- Avoiding social interactions
- Avoiding certain environments

- Constantly blaming yourself
- Not being able to engage in emotional intimacy

Can you think of some trauma responses that feel more unique to you and your family? You can start with reflecting on any stressful situations you've endured. How have you responded? How do your relatives generally respond to similar situations? How do you all tend to feel in those moments? And how do you cope?

The Keeper of Emotions

I'll tell a story from my own familial experience to illustrate the way in which trauma responses can be passed from one generation to the next. Like my grandmother, mother, and me, my papi, Rammy, has always been a keeper. But not a keeper of things. My father is a keeper of emotions. He holds on to his emotions until it seems his poor little heart is about to implode. My dad is a softy. Kind, gentle, humble to a fault, and an all-around loving human. Despite being pummeled with socialized messages about masculinity, messages particularly prevalent in the Latine community where machismo (a Spanish term meaning a strong, often toxic masculine pride) runs rampant, my dad kept his tenderness and his kind heart.

But when my dad isn't feeling well or has a challenging emotion, like fear or worry, he doesn't tell a soul. He holds it in until the issue passes. Whenever one of his family members is sick, for example, he worries. Intensely. We can see it in his eyes, but he'll never mention it. It is only after the illness is over, once things have gone back to normal, that we finally see my dad take a deep breath, or even cry, and release the fear he's been silently holding on to.

When I asked my dad why he never entertains discussions about the more challenging things he's going through or the fears he holds, he told me, "I don't want to place any burdens on my family." He doesn't want anyone else to feel the pain. So he *keeps* the emotion *for us*.

My dad has lived as an emotions keeper his entire life. His parents raised him to always be friendly, agreeable, and kind. Their lessons were beautiful, and I see so much light in my dad because of them. But when we place so much value on harmony and affability, there is little room for the expression of other, less tolerable emotional experiences. A common approach to problems on my dad's side of the family is "Let's not focus on the bad; everything will be OK." This sounded a bit like the concept of *toxic positivity*, which is when a person feels that they can only express positive emotions and therefore doesn't often display or discuss negative emotions and circumstances. When I asked my dad what he thought about that concept, he responded by saying that he sees it as more of a "realistic optimism." He says it's important to hold on to the faith that things will be OK and not entertain the possibility that something might go wrong. "It's how we protect our families from emotional burdens," he said. I get what he meant, especially because it had some cultural undertones that I understood personally. He meant that he will hold the negative emotions for his family, because as a father, he believes that to be his duty. This is a socialized message, and it's not an uncommon thing for a parent, particularly a father, to do in the Latine culture: to be the keeper of hard emotions on behalf of the people they love. But I also understood, from a psychological point of view, that a person can't always claim that everything is OK to make it so.

I understood that suppressed emotions don't disappear. They just find other ways to express themselves. For years, I saw how this realistic optimism, or perhaps disowning of hard emotions, was a definitive part of my father's formative years. Being raised to make space only for the good can challenge a person's ability to properly express the full range of emotions. There wasn't much room in my father's life to more outwardly express feelings of shame, fear, sadness, worry, or anxiety, which was also a generational norm for his era. And although he is more expressive and open about his feelings now that he's done some of this cycle-breaking work, for a large portion of his life, he struggled to let these emotions free.

My dad's instinct to hold on to heavy emotions, to keep them private in order to protect those around him from feeling "bad," is a reflection of love, but it is also his trauma response, and one that he unknowingly modeled for his children. I have always had a propensity to numb inconvenient emotions until the stressor passes. Through my work, I came to understand that this is a version of my dad's trauma response. I learned to become an emotions keeper, just like my father. This inherited trait has taken a long time and a ton of practice to release. I still care deeply for others, just not at my own expense. And I believe you can develop that standard too. Although this type of inheritance takes time and practice to undo, it can be healed. That's the main message I hope you hold on to here: that even when we have a long history of emotional weight, like my dad and I do, healing is possible. It has been for us, and it can be for you.

Breaking the Cycle: Your Intergenerational Trauma Tree

So where do we get started in doing the work? As I tell my clients, we can't look forward without looking back. And the same goes for you. The wounds you carry most likely span many generations. And although it won't be possible—or even necessary—to go back to the beginning of time to find the initial origins of the soul wounds of your family, whatever information you do know can still create enough of a map to help answer some critical questions for your healing journey. So let's take a moment to trace the origins of your pain through an Intergenerational Trauma Tree.

I'm going to ask you to draw a tree, from its roots up to its highest leaf. This tree will represent psychological, physical, spiritual, and cultural characteristics of people in your family and even your extended community. It will be made up of four equally important parts: the soil, the roots, the trunk, and the leaves. Each component contributes to the larger picture of you and your well-being by including the trauma of your ancestors as a part of your story. We want to pay close attention to developing each part of the tree and its corresponding characteristics so that when we zoom out, we see a clear picture of your intergenerational trauma narrative.

Tree mapping has been used extensively in narrative-based psychotherapy and other comparable therapies. When we map out a person's psychophysiospiritual (mind-body-spirit) experiences and the cultural messages they've internalized, we can gather a clearer image of what trauma may have been captured in the family unit. Here, we borrow from these therapeutic approaches to create an extended, more contextualized tree that offers the narratives of multiple generations, with the hope of gaining greater clarity into your family dynamics as a whole. Take your time with this exercise. This is a long line of histories and will take a moment to gather. Give yourself that extended moment.

We will start with the leaves, which signify each family member, then shift to the trunk, which is a reflection of their impact on you, then move down to the roots, which signify any beliefs that have become internalized, and finally go into the soil, which is reflective of the cultural norms that keep trauma in place for generations.

When you're ready, let's get started. Draw a tree on a sheet of paper, taking up all the space. Remember the four parts—the leaves, the trunk, the roots, and the soil—and be sure to leave plenty of space to write in each one. If you need a visual aid, take a look at the example I offer below. This should help you see how you'll start mapping out the tree. Take as much time as you need to create this tree and to breathe and release tension while completing it.

Intergenerational Trauma Tree

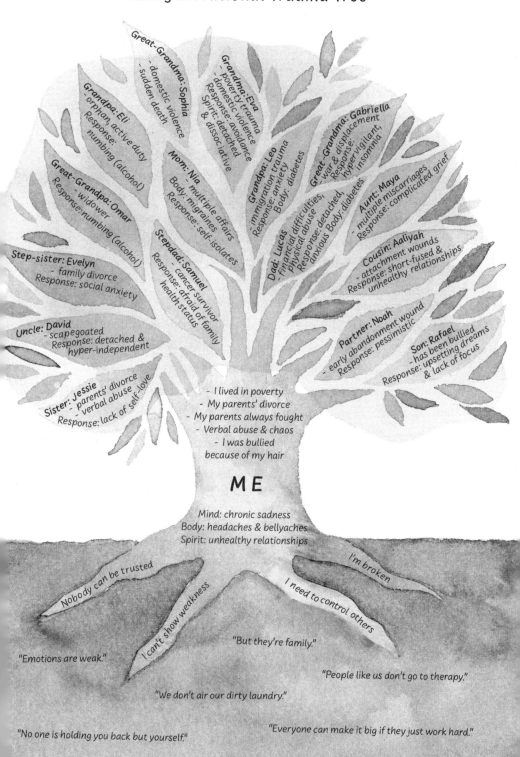

Great-Grandma: Sophia
- domestic violence
- sudden death

Grandpa: Eli
- orphan, active duty
Response:
numbing (alcohol)

Great-Grandpa: Omar
- widower
Response: numbing (alcohol)

Grandma: Eva
- poverty trauma
- domestic violence
Response: avoidance
Spirit: detached
& dissociative

Mom: Nia
- multiple affairs
Body: migraines
Response: self-isolates

Grandpa: Leo
- immigration trauma
Response: anxiety
Body: diabetes

Great-Grandma: Gabriella
- war & displacement
Response:
hypervigilant,
insomnia

Aunt: Maya
- multiple miscarriages
Response: complicated grief

Dad: Lucas
- financial difficulties,
physical abuse
Response: detached,
anxious Body: diabetes

Cousin: Aaliyah
- attachment wounds
Response: short-fused &
unhealthy relationships

Step-sister: Evelyn
- family divorce
Response: social anxiety

Stepdad: Samuel
- cancer survivor
Response: afraid of family
health status

Uncle: David
- scapegoated
Response: detached &
hyper-independent

Partner: Noah
- early abandonment wound
Response: pessimistic

Son: Rafael
- has been bullied
Response: upsetting dreams
& lack of focus

Sister: Jessie
- parents' divorce
- verbal abuse
Response: lack of self-love

- I lived in poverty
- My parents' divorce
- My parents always fought
- Verbal abuse & chaos
- I was bullied
because of my hair

ME

Mind: chronic sadness
Body: headaches & bellyaches
Spirit: unhealthy relationships

Nobody can be trusted

I'm broken

I need to control others

I can't show weakness

"But they're family."

"Emotions are weak."

"People like us don't go to therapy."

"We don't air our dirty laundry."

"No one is holding you back but yourself."

"Everyone can make it big if they just work hard."

"You have to take care of your younger siblings."

Now that your tree is drawn, let's start by filling in the leaves. The leaves signify each family member that you wish to be a part of your narrative. These can be people who are in direct descendant connection to you, like parents, grandparents, your children, and so on, and they can be people who are connected to you through one or two degrees of separation, like siblings, aunts, uncles, and cousins. If you have family that is either chosen or adopted or people who have had an extensive-enough connection to your life and lineage, feel free to add them as well. Emotional strain and resilience don't just come from the bloodline but from anyone who was close enough to have influence on your lived experience. This is your tree and your story, so make it yours.

The more family you can include, the better, but don't feel pressured to add people whom you don't have a historic report for. This tree is about visualizing information, so do your best to fill it in with the people whose stories you do have access to.

On each leaf, write the person's name, their relationship to you, any traumatic event that happened in that person's life, whatever personality characteristics they've adopted that were reflective of a trauma response, the ways their bodies responded (if they had any physical health issues, especially if they stemmed from chronic stress), and the ways their spirit captured these issues (through disconnection from self or others).

If it's helpful, some examples of traumatic events could be:

- Financial difficulties
- Major accidents
- Traumatic deaths
- Abuse (physical, emotional, sexual, financial, etc.)
- Identity bias or violence

Some examples of trauma responses could be what you wrote down before or these:

- Avoiding people, places, or things that trigger fear
- Having trouble setting proper boundaries
- Getting into high-risk situations
- Self-sabotaging
- People-pleasing in order to feel accepted or loved
- Numbing through mindless activities
- Oversharing or overexplaining in order to feel understood
- Lashing out when they're not feeling heard
- Denying their own reality (gaslighting themselves)
- Pushing love away because of struggles to accept love
- Overreading people, just in case other people could possibly hurt them
- Avoiding conflict
- Not speaking up for themselves

Common physical conditions with connections to trauma include:

- Metabolic conditions (e.g., diabetes, heart disease, hypertension, etc.)
- Autoimmune/inflammatory conditions (e.g., rheumatic diseases, fibromyalgia, irritable bowel syndrome, etc.)
- Other inflammatory conditions (e.g., headaches, chronic fatigue, muscle pain, etc.)

Common spirit-based disconnections could be:

- Lack of self-love
- Low sense of self-worth or self-esteem
- Inability to sustain healthy relationships
- Dissociating
- Feeling scapegoated
- Anything else that creates a disconnection from self and others

Common diagnosable mental health conditions associated with trauma responses could be the following:

- Depressive disorders (e.g., major depressive disorder, bipolar depression, etc.)
- Anxious disorders (e.g., obsessive-compulsive disorder [OCD], social anxiety, specific phobias, etc.)
- Post-traumatic stress disorder (PTSD)
- Attention deficit hyperactivity disorder (ADHD)
- Psychotic disorders (e.g., schizophrenia, delusional disorder, etc.)

Disclaimer: I believe there's a clinical utility in understanding how symptoms, taken together, can be seen as a condition to be treated by a mental health professional. I also find it useful that we name and call out any mental health challenges that have existed within our family units. However, it is important to understand that some labels can (1) be harmful, (2) be misinterpreted, and (3) don't allow us to see the complexity of traumatic experiences that have led a person to internalize these symptoms. Keep this point in mind as you add these to your intergenerational narrative.

Once you've considered all the layers of each leaf on your tree, we'll move on to the trunk. This part focuses more intently on you. Here, make a list of the ways in which the intergenerational strains of the individuals on the leaves have impacted you. These can be both direct and indirect experiences. An example of a direct experience is being explicitly told you aren't lovable by someone. An indirect experience would be learning that your grandmother was physically abusive to your mother. As a result, your mother became a very withdrawn person. So withdrawn, in fact, that she missed caring for your emotions in a way that you needed. So your grandmother's aggressive tendencies impacted you indirectly, or said another way, they impacted your mother's capacity for love and care, which then impacted how she cared for or missed caring for you.

Some additional examples of indirect impact are the following:

- A great-grandparent who was stuck in a pattern of people-pleasing and modeled that to their children, who modeled it to their children's children, who then modeled it to you. (So your great-grandparent's people-pleasing tendencies became a legacy that was passed down multiple generations and landed on you.)
- A grandmother who suffered with postpartum depression and couldn't emotionally connect to your father when he was a baby, and your father, who struggled to be emotionally attuned to you. (So the initial impact would have been on your father, but you suffered the intergenerational consequence of that unaddressed postpartum depression.)
- An older sibling who would physically hurt (you) their younger sibling, because they learned from your parents that when someone's angry, the appropriate behavior is to hit someone who's more vulnerable. (So the initial source of pain was your parents to your older sibling, but the secondary intergenerational target eventually became the younger sibling, you.)
- A parent who couldn't get loans because of their racial background, which led them to a debt they couldn't recover from and which then led to you not having enough resources growing up. (So the initial impact was on a parent, but you would have consequently suffered in traumatizing poverty thereafter.)

It can help if you start reflecting on specific experiences you had with each individual, again considering both the direct and indirect ways they have impacted you. To start, look at each leaf and ask yourself, "In what ways has *their* trauma contributed to the trauma that I've experienced?" This is where you get to start asking the popular question "What happened to you?" You can also ask yourself, "How did I get here?" "Who hurt me?" "What did they experience?" and "How was it that them not being able to break the cycle eventually caused me harm?"

Once you've completed your trunk, take a few deep breaths, because that was a lot. When you're ready, let's tend to the roots of this tree.

When we suffer, our minds create new realities, new beliefs, and new norms to help us cope. We change and develop a different way of being. I've changed, and so have you. And this part of the tree offers an opportunity for you to reflect on what truly has changed in you due to your family's experience of trauma. So here, you'll write on each root the different ways in which you've adopted limiting beliefs about yourself, others, and the world as a result of the distressful experiences you noted on the trunk. These are the internalized beliefs that maintain the cycle of trauma in you. Bringing awareness to them will help you in the later parts of your healing, to understand what beliefs need to be discarded. Some examples of these could be the belief that:

- "Nobody can be trusted."
- "People will only love me if I'm of use to them."
- "No matter how hard I try, I won't ever get far."
- "I'm broken, spoiled fruit."
- "I can't show any perceived sign of weakness."
- "If I show any vulnerability, I'm open to any threat."
- "I have to take care of everyone else first."
- "I need to control people; otherwise I feel like I'll lose control of myself."
- And any others that feel more personal to your lived experience

Take a moment to reflect on the beliefs you've personally held on to that are reflective of your wounds. Once you're done tending to the roots, it's time to dig in the dirt and move into the soil of your tree.

No tree system is complete without the soil that keeps it growing. You see, in society, we all internalize messages from our communities and the institutions that we're connected to, such as schools, religious centers, and the people in our culture. These institutions instill beliefs in us that can either propel us forward or keep cycles of trauma burgeoning in our communities. One example of a prominent cultural belief is that one shouldn't tell family business outside of family. It's a hard-and-fast rule for many communities. This belief can encourage harmful secret keeping at the individual and family level. So, when thinking about societal messages, I'd like for you to consider these kinds of cultural scripts that have driven common beliefs in your family members and in you.

Some examples of these messages can be:

- "You don't air your dirty laundry."
- "Even if they hurt you, they're still family, so you have to be nice to them."
- "You must respect your elders regardless of their behavior toward you."
- "We don't go to therapy; we solve our problems ourselves."
- "Depression isn't real; you have to just get up and shake it off."
- "Showing your emotions is a sign of weakness."
- "People outside of family can't be trusted."
- "Everyone has equal opportunity; nobody is holding you back but yourself."
- And any others that have been prominent in your life

Once you have completed the soil that surrounds the tree, the exercise is finished. Well, for now. You've completed a major part of a very difficult task, and so let's take a pause. At this point in your reflection, you're probably experiencing a lot of emotions. There may be a blend of anger and guilt and a sprinkle of sadness making its way into your heart. These responses are completely natural. And that's why we'll take a moment here to dive into some reflection with some guided writing.

Pause and Check In: How's Your Soul?

Grab your journal. Write about your process in completing your Intergenerational Trauma Tree. How did it make you *feel* (key word *feel*) to fill in every portion of your tree? Which parts were the most difficult? When did you find yourself hurting the most? Did anything make you feel sad or angry? Now, take time to consider where in your body these feelings appear. Do you feel them in your head? Your stomach? Your back? Last, take time to consider your spirit. How connected do you feel to yourself and to family after completing this practice?

What I'm really trying to get at here is: How is your soul? How do you feel in your mind, in your body, and in your spirit? This is my attempt at getting you to check in with yourself, fully and holistically. It's so important that we do this frequently throughout your journey. Because intergenerational trauma work is hard work. It is multidimensional, not just multigenerational. So, as you take in the next phases of this book, offer yourself a deeper check-in and ask, "How's my soul?" And if the word soul feels reminiscent of any religious or spiritual experiences that don't sit well with you, try using the modified question "How am I, really?" Once you do, offer yourself a few breaths to bring your mind-body-spirit back into a more neutral state. If it helps, pause here, and head over to this section's sound bath meditation to help you ground yourself.

What You've Learned So Far

This chapter contained a lot of information about biological transmissions of trauma, genes, and trauma responses across your lineage. There were a lot of heavy details, but you managed to apply what you learned to complete an Intergenerational Trauma Tree to map out your own intergenerational history. I hope you're proud of yourself for getting through this part of the journey. Now that you've completed all this, take some pauses and breaths, and focus on more reflection with the questions below. When you're ready, move into the next chapter, where you'll be taken through an understanding of your intergenerational nervous system.

REFLECTION QUESTIONS

What emotions come up when you think about the different ways
     your family's bodies have been genetically connected to stress?
How does it feel to take a deep dive into your lineage through your
     tree mapping exercise?
What are you looking forward to learning more about so far?

PART 2

There Are Layers to This

CHAPTER 6

Your Intergenerational Nervous System

A parent can't give you what they've never received.

—Lady, my sister

There is a branch of the human body's nervous system that is directly responsible for navigating interpersonal relationships. It helps us experience our connections to others in a way that feels safe and secure. Scientists have called this the *social nervous system.* It is a part of the human body that starts to develop in the womb and then rapidly in early childhood to help us form a relationship with our social environment. When a baby starts to connect with a caregiver's facial expressions and voice tones, they start to understand whether something is OK or wrong in the environment simply by observing that other person. With enough cues that the world around them is OK, that infant will start to feel safe and curious. But if a baby has a high level of emotional vulnerability and doesn't receive enough of those safety cues, they can start developing an overactive nervous system. When a parent suffers from an overactive nervous system and isn't able to connect with their baby in a way that helps them feel secure, they can contribute to their child developing an overactive nervous system, similar to their own.

The nervous system is structured to help you process stress temporarily and then release that stress so you can relax again. However, if you live with unresolved trauma, you will instead experience constant, elevated nervous system responses, which leave little room for stress release and relaxation. Because your mind stays hyperfocused on when the next danger will come, your nervous system rarely enters a calm state. That's how unresolved trauma can wear down your nervous system's ability to function properly.

Learning your way out of these cycles requires you to process how the trauma responses of your nervous system exist within you so that you can heal any fracturing that has taken place.

The Intergenerational Nervous System

We humans have a nervous system that discharges stress fairly similarly to how other mammals do it. Our nervous system is broken into three parts. The first is the sympathetic nervous system, which is the part of your nervous system that is alerted to a threat and prepares your mind and body for self-protection. It either prepares you to fight off the threat or to run away from it: the fight-or-flight response. The next is the dorsal vagal system. It's the part of the nervous system that is most implicated in emotional overwhelm. It's the shut-down system. When stress feels like it's too much to bear, the dorsal vagal system moves us into immobility and dissociation: the freeze response. At a more extreme level, it triggers profound bodily exhaustion and eventually leads to full body collapse: the fawn response. But in between these two parts of the nervous system, we have a very helpful and adaptive part, one that helps safely move us out of that protection response and keeps us from either entering a full shutdown or literally running for our lives. That third part of the nervous system is called the ventral vagal system, which you might remember from chapter 3's ventral vagal toning practice. It guards us from overestimating situations as threatening, keeps our emotions steady, and makes healthy connections to others more accessible. It's also the part of our nervous system that inhibits us from being impulsive when we are in fight or flight and instead offers us a greater range of actions to choose from. It is the part of the nervous system responsible for establishing and maintaining psychological safety. And psychological safety leaves more room for critical thinking, finding solutions, accessing memories, and creating safety for others. If we are not feeling safe in our own bodies, it's going to be very hard to live a life that's balanced and to create a safety container for those around us, including our children. Let's take a moment to increase your ventral vagal response now.

Sit comfortably in your seat. As you inhale, try filling up your lungs with air. Once your lungs are full, hold your breath for 2 seconds. Then, release your breath really slowly—for about 7 seconds. Repeat this process for a period of 5 minutes, because the nervous system typically requires that amount of time to enter a relaxation rhythm. Notice how your body responded to this reset. If you have achieved a calm state, that is the feeling of ease. But a nervous system that is stuck in a state of survival mode is not achieving this calm state with enough frequency. It is, instead, stuck in a spiral of hyper- or hypoarousal. If you don't feel calm after this exercise, just know that it takes a number of repetitions of these exercises to start seeing their effect. You may not feel the impact right away and that's OK.

Let's bring this concept of an unsettled nervous system back to Brooklyn's multigenerational home. Brooklyn never felt contained and safe. In her home, everyone felt the tension of someone else's stress. By her description, I understood that they were all living in survival mode. And this survival mode was further perpetuating traumas in Brooklyn's family. Brooklyn's mother and aunt had internalized their own mother's elevated emotional states, and by the time we began our work together, so had Brooklyn. When one negative thing happened to one family member, all of them would share the stress, which would contribute to the chaos in their shared home. Her mother and grandmother would yell at each other: the fight response. Brooklyn and her aunt would shut down and disengage: the fawn response. Each of them had different types of survival mode responses to their family's collective stress. And each of these responses was a reflection of an emotional destabilization, meaning their emotions were difficult for them to control.

This contagion effect of multiple destabilized nervous systems is what I call an *intergenerational nervous system*, a term you might remember from the last chapter.

To add a layer to this dynamic, Brooklyn's mother and aunt were twins, and so Brooklyn's grandmother, her mother, her aunt, and Brooklyn had all existed in one body at one point in time. Miraculous, right? When her grandmother was pregnant, all four of them were exposed to the same stressors and a similar genetic encoding. And although they now existed in separate bodies, they were still profoundly connected to one another. Their intergenerational nervous system was reinforced through their behavior, their deep genetic ties, and the pervasive emotional destabilization that defined their shared family home. The experiences of our ancestors produce something like a fingerprint, imprinting unique neural patterns on our brains through the generations. Psychologists suspect that these fingerprints contribute to the subsequent development of psychiatric conditions and that the biological transmission of these imprints could help us understand certain temperaments and susceptibility to conditions like anxiety, for example. Behavioral difficulties, cognitive problems, and other psychological issues have also been observed transmitting down genetic lines. Furthermore, where there was either a compromise in trust, dishonesty, lack of openness in the family, or relationship problems, there was a notable difference in expressions of descendants of trauma.

Dr. LeManuel Lee Bitsóí, a member of the Navajo Nation, has directed a number of genome science studies at Harvard University's Center of Excellence in Genome Sciences. He has added to our current understanding of epigenetic transmission through his work, which aims to uncover the ways in which intergenerational trauma and historical trauma have been a contributing cause of both mental and physical illnesses in Native American families. Scientific studies are additionally revealing the multiple ways in which epigenetic modification can even compromise organ systems (e.g., the brain, heart, or kidneys), thereby influencing how these structures develop and function. Multiple connections exist between stress and the well-being of those impacted by stress, and multiple areas of scientific inquiry are helping us get a clearer biological picture of the impact of unmetabolized trauma and the mind-body fracturing that can happen across generations.

Although several worldwide studies in recent decades have looked closely at the genetic load of both mental and physical illnesses, the most telling evidence of how these experiences get transferred from one generation to the next comes from the stories of the families themselves. It comes from the layers reflected in your Intergenerational Trauma Healing Assessment and your Intergenerational Trauma Tree, which is why we get into those layers here first. Because, if you dig deep enough, you will see that families have carried stories that speak to how intergenerational trauma has been at the center of their pain. There are details in our stories that are more nuanced and complex than any scientific area can study. There are trauma responses that have been recycled and require us to unravel the layers, bit by bit. And when we do, we notice that many families, including our own, are holding on to these intergenerational trauma triggers that continue to get passed down, time and again.

Intergenerational Triggers

When a person's trauma symptoms have been detained, meaning when a person is experiencing chronic signs of trauma, these symptoms cause what's known as a traumatic retention. But your brain is smart, and it hides this tension masterfully behind your psychological defenses. This coping mechanism is preprogrammed in you to help you continue living your life after experiencing a trauma. But sometimes the hidden strain of the past is unlocked by a trigger, and it places your nervous system back into a fight, flight, freeze, or fawn response. It teleports you back in time to the traumatic event.

Triggers can be internal emotional signals (e.g., a loss of self-control, feeling abandoned, experiencing shame, etc.) and external sensory signals (e.g., the sight of an accident, the smell of someone's cologne, a loud noise, etc.). When a memory of the past is unlocked before you've properly healed from it, the experience can cause you to tense up. These triggers activate memories and evoke a reaction in your nervous system. Each person has only a certain capacity to handle difficult emotions, and the tolerance for elevated emotions is unique to that individual. Your tolerance is determined by a number of factors. The most notable here is what I call your *intergenerational window of tolerance*.

Your window of tolerance is the emotional space within which you are comfortable and feel safe. In this window, you can deal with daily stressors, work through solutions in life and relationships, and feel relatively balanced. But when you are pushed beyond your emotional limit, a hyperarousal response (where you experience high energy, hypervigilance, anxiety, anger, restlessness, agitation, and irritability) or hypoarousal response (where you experience withdrawal, numbing, shame, depression, and shutdown) can be triggered. Now, your intergenerational window of tolerance is reflective of your own emotional limitations *layered with* the emotional limitations of the people who came before you.

When a parent has a nervous system that is chronically in a stress response, their children are then more susceptible to having a similar nervous system structure—a biological inheritance of emotional vulnerability. Biologically, their children could already experience greater discomfort with difficult emotions than children whose parents do not experience that chronic stress response. Additionally, a parent models their emotional capacities—or incapacities—to their children, unconsciously teaching their children how to respond to stress. They also model their window of tolerance for their children, who then adopt a similar window of tolerance for themselves. This can be a bit complex to understand, so let me help illustrate it with an example from the therapy room.

I once had a client, Zuri, whose father had experienced trauma. As a result, when even the most minor thing would happen, he would enter a state of hypoarousal, or emotional shutdown. He had a critically small window of tolerance, meaning that he had very little capacity to handle stressful situations. For him, anything beyond a mild stressor would cause a major emotional shutdown. This response was triggered by both his predisposed emotional vulnerabilities and his own past traumas that made it difficult for him to tolerate minimal stress well. Therefore, he had a hard time staying calm and focused when put under pressure and would easily withdraw, shifting into a fawn/shutdown response where he relied on alcohol to numb his overcharged emotions. This chain of behavior was the modeled stress response that my client had observed since infancy, and over time, it had become the behavioral response she developed to cope with her own stress.

My client had already been born with a vulnerability to high stress. She was even told that as a baby, she was extremely hard to calm and console, and that the smallest thing would cause her to burst into long bouts of crying. Fast-forward to when she was a kid, whenever she felt overwhelmed—taken out of her own window of tolerance—she would shift into hypoarousal, just like her father. Her nervous system response defaulted to both the one she was predisposed to genetically and the one she saw being modeled by her dad. She was embodying a generational inheritance of emotional vulnerability, feeling easily exhausted and dissociating, and also learning that the way to cope with having a narrowed window of tolerance was to fawn or shut down.

Once this response was triggered, my client wouldn't speak to anyone and would self-isolate. But when she became a parent herself, she was dismayed to see her own children displaying a similar coping response to the one she had inherited from her father. She was witnessing a cycle of diminished intergenerational windows of tolerance, meaning a cycle of diminished stress tolerance. My client's children offered a mirror into her own soul. She wanted to be a cycle breaker and to pass down a better legacy to her children and future generations. This meant that together, we needed to dig into the intergenerational nervous system responses reflected in her family and expand her window of tolerance in this generation so that she would then have an opportunity to model this skill to her children.

This is a task for you to consider as well. In our families of origin, we each learned how to respond to stressors in our own lives by observing our family members and caregivers. This is the process of building an overactive intergenerational nervous system. Families inherit certain stress responses from each other. Each family and each person within a family will have their own version of what this looks like. Your family's intergenerational nervous system won't look identical to anyone else's. It will, instead, look like the unique trauma responses reflected in your Intergenerational Trauma Tree. And you will notice that there is a way in which the leaves feed the trunk, or that the soil feeds the roots, and that the whole tree's ecosystem is flowing in a pain cycle. At the heart of that cycle are a set of intergenerational nervous system responses that have not yet been disrupted. Learning what these are can help you shift those generational responses into healthier ones.

Some other examples of intergenerational nervous system responses could be:

- The learned survival response of staying quiet (you became stuck in freeze mode) around parents whose trauma response was to yell when under stress (they were stuck in fight mode)
- The learned behavior of withdrawing from a situation (you became stuck in fawn/shut-down mode) when an elder would become physically abusive (they were stuck in fight mode)
- The learned response to always scream to defend yourself (you became stuck in fight mode) because adults in your life were constantly blaming you and verbally berating you (they were also stuck in fight mode)
- The learned survival response to flee situations when uncomfortable (you became stuck in flight mode) because no one listened to you and people tended to avoid problems (they were also stuck in flight mode)
- What others might you add to the list that feel more aligned with your experience?

I've always been fascinated by the multiple ways in which trauma responses can show up in one family line. But it was when I started to review my own family tree that I began to understand this concept more deeply and on a personal level. I saw a pattern of responses my family members all presented. My mother has mostly been stuck in fight mode. She fights tooth and nail when she is pushed beyond her emotional limits. My father has a default flight mode. He holds in his emotions and settles away from the conflict. My sister took on a similar nervous system response as my father. She has defaulted to fleeing from conflict for most of her life. And I mirrored my mother's trauma response, so for me, fight mode was familiar and comfortable.

Although we had variable default nervous system responses, one common thread among us was that we had a family that was collectively hyperaroused. It was especially apparent when we were all together and our individual nervous systems started feeding off each other, forming an unsettled intergenerational nervous system. We spent decades absorbing and amplifying each other's trauma responses. That is, until my sister and I decided to be cycle breakers. When we learned to restructure our responses and open up space for my parents to do the same, we began to heal as a unit.

It is incredibly hard to shift from our deeply programmed trauma responses to more constructive behaviors. I speak from personal and professional experience. But I think it goes without saying that if you don't mobilize toward trauma disruption, you will find yourself living with the same trigger response inheritance for years. Forever, if you never find a way to address it. If you don't tend to your trauma, your legacy will be an inheritance of an unsettled intergenerational nervous system, a narrow intergenerational window of tolerance, and a set of intergenerational trigger responses for yourself, for your children, and for their children. This is why cycle breaking is such urgent work.

Intergenerational Memories

No one *wants* to get triggered or to stay in intergenerational trigger responses. More often than not, triggers drop into your life unannounced and from a wide range of internal and external sources. That's because intergenerational triggers include different, buried recollections that make up the vast network of *intergenerational memories*. Trigger memories can send you to another place and time, sometimes even to a memory beyond your own lifetime.

Let's take, for example, my client Leon. When Leon's grandfather was twenty years old, before he had any children, he suffered a bad beating from a stranger. He was left with a concussion and some bruised ribs. And he was also left with a scent memory. Apparently, his attacker had had a cup of coffee before the attack and the scent of it left a memory imprint. For the rest of his life, whenever Leon's grandfather smelled coffee, it triggered him, sending him back to the moment when he was attacked. He would feel ill and would shut down emotionally, his body preparing him to receive another beating, even though there was no threat present.

Here's where it gets interesting. Leon's mother, born years after the attack, found the smell of coffee to be repulsive just like her father had, and Leon himself felt his stomach turn when he smelled it. Three generations of memories were activated, triggered by the scent of coffee, which had been present in one traumatic incident decades in the past.

This may sound fantastical, but both scent memory and the genetic transmission of those memories are a well-studied phenomenon. Smell can be a particularly strong memory connector when linked to our childhood memories. Many survivors of childhood sexual abuse report how the scents in the home where the abuse happened are stamped in their memory. Well into their adulthood, they say how triggering it can be to be around those smells. Scent imprints itself deep into your brain. The sense of smell is especially linked to memory because scents take a direct route to the limbic system of the brain. Given its direct ride to the center of the brain into a system connected to your nervous system responses, scent is a powerful memory retriever. Further still, studies have shown that scent-trauma pairing has a multigenerational effect and that the sensitivity to specific smells transcends generations. Fascinating, right?

There are so many memories that you don't have immediate access to. And some of that may be for good reason. It's that protective function of your mind I mentioned earlier in this chapter, to obscure some painful memories, and it helps you conserve mental energy. This is a coping mechanism that helps you function after a traumatic event. However, a cache of inherited memories are stored in your DNA, waiting for you to access them—memories that, should they be retrieved, could help you construct a more comprehensive understanding of how you got here and how you can heal.

Types of intergenerational memories include:

- **Cellular Memory**—the memory of multigenerational stress that is carried in your cells and genes. Our cells are so smart. They keep a record of what happens to us and even what happened before us. The gene expressions we have in our cells that reflect high levels of stress and get triggered more easily by stressful circumstances are reflective of this type of memory. Our cells know that we come from our parents' stressed bodies, and they retain that stress memory within them, reacting and responding to both the memories of stress of the past and to the stressors of the present.
- **Procedural Memory**—the memory of emotional strain that is carried in your body, namely in your brain and nervous system. These memories can be reignited by something that happens in our lives. An example of this is the smell of coffee that made its way down generations of Leon's family. Our senses—our capacity to smell, see, taste, touch, and hear—all attach to our memories. This is why when we are triggered, we get taken back by way of our senses, meaning by way of something in our current environment that we smell, see, taste, touch, or hear that reminds us of the past.
- **Intuitive Memory**—the inner knowing that something has happened in your lineage and has led to some grief in your own soul. Your gut feeling is a memory. Your déjà vu moments are memories. Your dreams are reflections of your memories. These are all locked into your intuition and help you develop an inner knowing beyond your conscious thought.

Triggers and trauma memories are interwoven into so many layers of the psyche that they can sneak up on you when you least expect them. But your healing journey is about expanding your self-knowledge and then using that new level of inner knowing as a tool for your healing.

Before we move on, let me ask: How does this all sit with you? Do any of these memory types spark a thought or emotion in you? If so, this could be a great moment to pause and journal. It can also be a moment to simply sit in silence and notice how you feel. Remember that when you sit and meditate, it's always a good idea to take a few deep breaths. Once you're ready, let's move on to this chapter's exercise.

Breaking the Cycle: Widening Your Intergenerational Window of Tolerance

Expanding your window of tolerance moves you away from triggers and closer to safety and connection. It does this by boosting how much stress you can tolerate at any given point in time. Our goal is to increase your capacity to tolerate stress so that it doesn't get planted in your soul and become a burden you carry around for life. To achieve this takes daily practice, and many repetitions, but in the long term it is worth it because it will help your nervous system relax more rapidly and more frequently.

For this chapter's practice, I would like to focus on expanding your safe zone. Let's introduce a modified, intergenerationally informed emotional freedom technique (EFT) to your daily routine. EFT is a mind-body practice that stimulates acupressure points through tapping and has been known to help with reducing symptoms related to stress, anxiety, depression, and trauma. For this practice, we will borrow the *om* sound from Sanskrit, an ancient and classical language of India. Om is considered to be the most powerful of all mantras and emits sound vibrations that directly connect to our nervous system's relaxation branch: the ventral vagal nerve, which you may remember from our discussions of the ventral vagal nervous system. For this inter-generational EFT practice, follow these prompts:

- Find a comfortable seat in a place that feels safe. If you can sit outside, even better, since we are focusing on grounding you during this practice. If you prefer to practice in the safe space you developed within the *Getting Ready to Do the Work* section in chapter 1 (see page 19), you can go there now.
- Once you're settled, find your breath and deepen it.
- Increase the time spent on both the inhale (approximately 5 seconds) and exhale (approximately 7 seconds).
- With your next inhale, bring to mind an image of yourself feeling cool, calm, and collected.
- With your next exhale, breathe out with the mantra sound *om*, breathing healing energy into this image of yourself in your safe zone.
- With the following inhale, bring to mind the image of an ancestor who didn't have access to healing tools to expand their own window of tolerance, and to whom you would like to send some healing vibrations.
- With your next exhale, release the mantra sound *om*, and imagine breathing out loving and healing energy onto your ancestor.
- Now bring your breath into a neutral rhythm, breathing as you normally would.
- Cup your hands and take your pointer, middle, and ring fingers to tap gently five times onto the meridian points listed below. With each tap, remember to breathe.
  - Tap the top of your head, your crown: your governing vessel that travels along your back, which is most connected to your nervous system.

- Tap the inner corners of your eyebrows: your bladder meridian, which is most connected to experiences of fear and troubling memories.

- Tap the outer corners of your eyes: your gallbladder meridian, which is most connected to the experience of emotional repression.

- Tap right under your eyes: your stomach meridian, which is most connected to the experience of despair.

- Tap right under your nose: also your governing vessel, which is also connected to your nervous system.

- Tap your chin area: your central vessel, which connects to all other functions of your mind and body.

- Tap right above your collarbone, on each side: your kidney meridian, which connects mostly to shame

- Tap under your arms (your armpits): your spleen meridian, which is mostly connected to apathy and disgust.

- Tap the outer meaty part of your hands: your small intestine meridian, which is most connected to denial and numbing.

- To finalize this practice, we are going back full circle, so bring your hands down to your sides.
- Deepen your breath once again.
- Increase the time spent on both the inhale (5 seconds) and exhale (7 seconds).
- With your next inhale, bring to mind an image of yourself feeling cool, calm, and collected.
- With your next exhale, breathe out with the mantra sound *om*, breathing healing energy into this image of yourself in your safe zone.
- With the following inhale, bring to mind the image of an ancestor who didn't have access to healing tools to expand their safe zone, and to whom you would like to send some healing vibrations to.

- With your next exhale, breathe out with the mantra sound *om*, breathing healing energy onto your ancestor.
- Now bring your breath into a neutral rhythm, breathing as you normally would.
- Send appreciation to your ancestors for being present for this offering and to yourself for taking the time to disrupt the trauma sequence captured in your nervous system.

What You've Learned So Far

In this chapter, we covered one of the main transporters of intergenerational trauma: your intergenerational nervous system. We went through the different ways in which the trauma responses held in one generation get transferred through nervous system responses down the family line. That preprogrammed nervous system response can be a lot to take in, so give yourself a moment to digest this information, and perhaps return to your intergenerational EFT tapping practice for more nervous system relaxation. As an added way to settle your intergenerational nervous system, you can dive into this section's sound bath meditation for more grounding. When you're ready, transition into this chapter's reflection questions and head over to the next chapter, where we will cover your intergenerational inner child.

REFLECTION QUESTIONS

How was it for you to learn about the multiple layers of your intergenerational nervous system?

What intergenerational triggers and trauma responses did you find to exist in your family and community?

What came to mind as you engaged in the tapping technique as a cycle-breaking practice?

CHAPTER 7

Your Intergenerational Inner Child

I became what I am today at the age of twelve.

—Khaled Hosseini

The quality of your early childhood relationships, particularly those with your caregivers, builds the foundation for how you're able to relationally attach to others. If those formative relationships were safe and supportive, then you were better able to build a secure attachment style and healthy trust, and you are able to maintain closeness in relationships. Alternatively, if these critical years were unsafe and you weren't provided with a supportive environment, you likely developed an insecure attachment style and suffered an inner child wound instead. As a result, every relationship you have will run the risk of being marked by versions of the same emotional injuries you sustained. That also means that if you're able to learn to build safety, trust, and secure bonds through your own healing, you can help undo the emotional injuries that happened in your childhood. Let's take this moment to understand the remnants of childhood stress and the protocol for healing intergenerational inner child wounds.

Childhood Stress: How the Transmission Continues

We humans are hardwired for connection. We need to feel a sense of belonging, attachment, and safety around others. We instinctively seek experiences to help us develop connection from the day we are born. As babies, we cry when we need comforting. Biologically, the cry signals an adult to come hold us in the safety of a hug and give us a tender smile to indicate everything is all right. The message that this sends our developing brain and nervous system is: "If I need someone, they will be responsive. And so, I can count on others."

A rhythm develops between children and their caretakers in those early years. Let's say that as an infant, you were left in your crib while an adult went to get your milk. Then, that adult came back to the crib with your warm milk, fed you, smiled at you, and burped you so that you could experience comfort. They left, then they came back. They took care of your needs and gave you a smile of assurance and safety. You could then rest and digest, the basic mechanism of a settled nervous system. You registered that your caregivers could be trusted, they could be a signal for a safe world, and they could bring you the comfort that you couldn't independently obtain for yourself. That consistent supply of attention is the basis for a secure attachment, the type of relational connection style that occurs as a result of feeling protected by your caregivers and knowing that you can depend on them to show up for you. Even if you can't remember these interactions, they had a profound impact on your development.

For children who grew up in homes with trauma, the pattern can be vastly different. The connection between caregiver and child may be muddled by abuse, neglect, drug use, mental illness, codependency, toxicity, poor emotional attunement, or disconnection. Under those circumstances, attachment cannot find a secure base. Instead, those families become stuck in trauma loops.

A baby develops reciprocal patterns of expressions when interacting with their caregiver. If the adult reflects positive facial expressions, the baby can rest and explore their world with gentle curiosity. But if the facial expressions are not responsive, as when, for example, a parent is dissociating and misses the baby's need for engagement, the baby notices the shift immediately and makes repeated attempts to regain the parent's attention and care. This ongoing monitoring of a caregiver's availability is exhausting and eventually leads a baby into emotional shutdown. In that scenario, we have a parent who is emotionally stunted and a baby who, for the sake of survival, has learned to shut down in the same way. This means that persistent and unexamined trauma symptoms in adults can create early emotional fracturing in their children. This, in turn, contributes to the development of an insecure child, a child whose ability to trust others has been compromised.

Fast forward a few years and that insecure child will develop a greater need for validation. However, since their parent is still likely overwhelmed by their own trauma, they'll be too preoccupied to attend to their child in ways that help build a secure foundation. This sends the message that their child is "too much" and "hard to love." And if unattended, these messages become internalized and create inner child wounds that start during these critical periods of development but last a lifetime.

Critical Periods

Certain moments during human development are what developmental scientists consider to be critical periods of growth. Your time in the womb is one such critical period, where you are developing all the vital organs you will need to live, and the first few years of life are another, because they help you establish the foundations for social connection.

It is during both of these critical periods that most stress responses become hardwired in the nervous system and brain. When a baby hears loud yelling noises in the home, their tiny nervous system goes on alert and their trigger responses surface: rapid heartbeat, shallow breaths, constricted digestion, dilated pupils, sweat, and muscle tension. The baby is in a fight, flight, freeze, or fawn response. The baby's amygdala, a primary emotion center of the brain, is also on high alert. Stress hormones are flooding their little body. If this happens often enough, their developing bodies can become stuck in a state of stress.

Now let's consider where the frequent yelling noises are coming from. If the yelling in the baby's home is a pattern, then it is very likely coming from an adult who is in a state of unrest. They, too, might be living with an inflamed nervous system, one that is unsettled. Already, that makes two people embodying a high level of toxic stress. Just like that, the stress has become intergenerational. The adult who couldn't properly regulate their emotions just contributed to the faulty regulation of their child's nervous system. Science tells us that without addressing that inherited stress, when that baby grows up, they will pass down the same stress to their children. And around and around we go.

Now, some stress is essential for normal development. Managing stress is adaptive and we have a nervous system that is built to effectively manage tolerable stress. However, a body that lives in persistent trauma is a body that has endured too much stress. It has lived under an ongoing, unrelenting layer of emotional strain. When stress reaches these levels, the person experiencing it will find it harder to move that energy out of their body. As a result, your body becomes a depository for that harmful emotional energy. If that stress happens very early in life, it develops into a wound that follows you into adulthood. This is a typical symptom of adverse childhood experiences.

Intergenerational Adverse Experiences

One of the strongest pieces of supporting research that we have on the role of traumatic stress in our society comes from the adverse childhood experiences (ACEs) study by the Centers for Disease Control and Prevention (CDC). The ACEs study started in the 1990s in California and surveyed over 17,000 health maintenance organization (HMO) members from Southern California about experiences in childhood that produced a lasting negative impact in people's lives. The core findings led researchers to focus on the experiences of parental incarceration, substance use, domestic abuse, loss of a parent through divorce or death, sexual trauma, emotional and physical neglect, mental illness in the family, and the experiencing or witnessing of violence. When it was first introduced, it offered a form of validation that had long been missing in the therapy room. The initial study had shortcomings, as it was not inclusive of diverse experiences of people from multiple cultural identities, nor did it account for variable experiences outside these core areas of focus. Still, exploring a person's adverse childhood experiences in relation to that seminal study remains a key therapy conversation starter for most trauma survivors.

My client Leon and I began discussing his adverse childhood experiences during one of our initial sessions. We decided to dive deeper into the ACEs questionnaire together. The original ACEs study includes ten questions about childhood adversity and allows the person or clinician to tally them at the end. Scores on the questionnaire can range from zero to ten, with zero meaning there were no incidents of childhood adversity and ten meaning there were a total of ten notable categories of childhood adversities that the person suffered through. As Leon learned about ACEs, he began expressing how this new way of seeing his childhood traumas gave him a sense of relief. And yet, while the questionnaire did help us fill in some gaps of knowledge about what happened to Leon in his own childhood, it didn't help us fill in the full story. Not only were harmful aspects of his upbringing not reflected in the original ACEs questionnaire, and even the subsequently modified versions we then had access to, but the questionnaire also failed to capture his intergenerational history. And because evidence shows that a parent's emotional instability can lead to maltreatment that then influences a child's emotional and behavioral functioning, we needed to shed light on that layer of his childhood adversity as well.

Leon and I started developing a more comprehensive, more personalized, and more intergenerational ACEs version in the hope that we could tell his whole story in a way that incorporated his family's history too. It is from my work with Leon and with other clients who felt this same limitation that I decided I would work on my Intergenerational Adverse Experiences Questionnaire. This assessment allowed my clients to fill in the gaps and make their recollection of adverse experiences more layered and nuanced.

Three core areas became the focus: (1) What happened to you? (2) What happened before you? and (3) What happened around you? These questions allowed us an opportunity to speak not only to what happened directly to my clients but also to what had happened indirectly (within their families and communities) that also had contributed to the adversity in their lives. Although I left a lot of room for us to codevelop what the Intergenerational Adverse Experiences Questionnaire could look like for each individual client, we started with a focus on a few themes. My clients selected the experiences from this list that made most sense to them, based on their recollection of experiences. As you read these, I would encourage you to do the same. Select the items on the list that connect to your generational experiences. Unlike the original ACEs questionnaire, we will not tally the responses and give you a number to focus on, although for research and data collection purposes, scoring can be an important tool to consider. However, for the purposes of the healing protocol we are following here, tallying up scores can distract us from the more comprehensive and nuanced story that each of your answers can offer. We will instead treat each item on the list as a conversation starter for you to reflect on. So, as you read, select the ones that make sense, and if you wish, journal about each item to expand your reflections on each individual experience. Do so with the understanding that the "What Happened Before You?" and "What Happened Around You?" portions of this questionnaire in no way excuse the harmful behaviors of what happened to those who didn't break the cycle before you or the harmful behaviors, beliefs, practices, and structural harm imposed by the institutions around you that have facilitated a trauma injury. It is simply there to help you understand the layers of the pain and trauma that are all a part of your history.

What Happened to You? (Direct Childhood Adversity)
- I wasn't shown love and affection.
- I was verbally or emotionally abused.
- I was chronically invalidated.
- I was physically beaten.
- I was sexually molested.
- My parents had an unhealthy separation or divorce.
- My family had domestic disputes.
- A loved one died prematurely or violently.
- We were displaced from our home.
- I had to or was forced to emigrate from a familiar place.
- I experienced medical trauma.
- I experienced financial poverty.
- My caregivers were imprisoned.
- I was persecuted or oppressed based on my cultural identity.
- Someone had a persistent mental health challenge in our home.
- Someone had a persistent physical illness in our home.
- Someone close to me suffered from an addiction.
- Any other instances that felt *personally* traumatic

What Happened Before You? (Intergenerational Childhood Adversity)

- My parents/grandparents/family/ancestors weren't shown love and affection.
- They were verbally or emotionally abused.
- They were chronically invalidated.
- They were physically beaten.
- They were sexually molested.
- They had parents who had a tragic separation or divorce.
- Adults in their family had domestic disputes.
- Their loved one died prematurely or violently.
- They were displaced from their home.
- They were forced to emigrate due to dire conditions.
- They experienced medical trauma.
- They experienced financial poverty.
- Their caregivers were imprisoned.
- They experienced persecution or oppression based on their cultural identity.
- Someone had a persistent mental health challenge in their home.
- Someone had a persistent physical illness in their home.
- Someone suffered an addiction in their home.
- Any other instances that felt *intergenerationally* traumatic

What Happened Around You? (Community or Societal Collective Adversity)

- We suffered a global pandemic.
- We had to live in fear of being violently targeted because of a marginalized identity.
- We embodied harmful cultural values that were normalized and allowed for the perpetuation of further trauma.
- We were survivors of cultural genocide.
- We suffered ongoing and pervasive cultural oppression.

- We were forced to assimilate to a different culture and language.
- We had to witness a community member(s) being terrorized or killed.
- Our lives were invalidated or targeted systemically.
- We were adversely impacted by a natural disaster.
- Any other instances that felt collectively traumatic

Leon found this modification of the ACEs questionnaire to be more validating and eye-opening. Through his own recollections, he was able to see how cultural messages about corporal punishment ran rampant through his family and community. He reflected on how this physical discipline had been normalized in his community (collective/cultural— what happened culturally around Leon—which answers the question "What happened around you?"), how his father suffered severe beatings by his own father's fists and mother's belt (intergenerational— what happened intergenerationally in Leon's family—which answers the question "What happened before you?"), and how he couldn't escape the physical and psychological pain his parents then transmitted to him (individual—how Leon directly suffered traumas—which answers the question "What happened to you?"). He was able to develop a more comprehensive view of his traumatic childhood experiences that, though painful to reflect on, helped him shed some of the heavy weight he carried.

As we move through all these layers of painful experiences, the question at the heart of the modified ACEs questionnaire becomes "What happened to you *through the generations*?" This question looks beyond your own childhood and also focuses on both the inner child wounds of your ancestors and the systemic influences that have perpetuated trauma in your lineage. This exercise becomes an exploration of the ways in which your family's past traumas can overwhelm your soul in the present. The point is not necessarily to build empathy for anyone who didn't do the work to break this cycle themselves (either because they lacked resources or motivation or because they were intentional about causing harm), although empathy does also come up for some cycle breakers. Instead, the point of this exercise is to know the full story of your trauma in order to help you heal from it as fully as humanly possible.

As a clinician, I would combine the information collected from this Intergenerational Adverse Experiences Questionnaire, the Intergenerational Trauma Healing Assessment, and the Intergenerational Trauma Tree to lay out the full picture of what my clients and I would be working on. Although this may sound like a daunting and heavy task, I was oftentimes met with motivation and curiosity about what our next steps would be in helping my clients release their pain. This can be a healthy point in your reading to pause, reflect, and write about what this all means to *you*, specifically and intergenerationally. Take a look back at all this data collection you've engaged in so far. How is it sitting with you? What are some patterns you can carve out from what you've written down so far? And since we are about to dive into your inner child with greater intention, how has your inner child taken in all these wounded experiences? Because this can be emotionally taxing for you to do, this would also be a good moment to take a few nourishing deep breaths before hopping into the next section.

Their Inner Child Becomes Your Inner Child

It's common for trauma victims to become emotionally stuck at the age at which our safety and connection were compromised. This is the age when our sensitivities were heightened and we developed an acute awareness that we were no longer in a safe or stable environment. This is the age that is marked by what psychologists call the *inner child wound*, a childhood-derived psychological weight that you carry.

Your inner child is a reflection of your suppressed childhood emotions that never got a chance to be fully felt and effectively managed. This suppression most often comes back up later in life. You may notice that you have a deep fear that someone, anyone, might abandon you. This may stem from an experience in childhood when you felt abandoned by a caregiver. Or perhaps you have low self-esteem, people-pleasing tendencies, and trouble setting boundaries, which coincide with a history of being neglected emotionally or physically as a child. It could also be that you feel insecure, an experience that has a connection to feeling that you couldn't trust the adults around you. Or perhaps you default to feeling guilty about most things, which may be the result of being blamed and scapegoated in your childhood. In all these experiences, childhood pain left an emotional impression in you as you aged into adulthood. The impressions left by these experiences don't go away on their own. Instead, they pour into your adult friendships, romantic connections, careers, and relationships with your children. That is, until you learn to fill the void, attend to your inner child, and re-parent yourself.

Everyone has an inner child, including your parents. If they weren't able to experience a healthy childhood, they too developed these wounds, which would lead them to (1) internalize negative ideas about their self-worth, and (2) pass on those same ideas to you. But how does that happen? Well, most of it is done through modeling. For example, if when your parents were children, their emotions were suppressed in the service of others, they would have demonstrated a habit of people-pleasing. As a child, you may have seen them over-appease others and then you soaked up those characteristics that they exhibited in relationships. You internalized these relationship qualities as your own. This is an example of an intergenerational inner child transmission, which is a childhood emotional wound modeled by your parents and inherited by you.

In addition to modeling, family members can also impose direct harm on you that also contributes to your intergenerational inner child transmission. For example, some families physically abuse their children for generations. Let's say that your great-grandparents learned that the way to keep their child, your grandmother, in line was by physically punishing her. That strategy created an inner child wound in her, but it also created a model for how she would then punish her own child (your father). That's how the cycle continued. Physical punishment is an example of what a caregiver *does to* their child that keeps the cycle going.

Another way an inner child transmission is perpetuated is through what caregivers *didn't do*, like offer emotional support. For example, if as a child, your father didn't receive emotional validation from his parents, then he won't intuitively know to check in on your emotions either. He never learned that children's emotions need validation. So that emotional neglect that you've felt so deeply was also prominent in him. This offers no excuse for a child's needs to be neglected, but it offers us an intergenerational lens by which to see how emotional neglect cycles continue.

Both what was done to you (like physical punishment) and what was not given to you (like lack of emotional validation) could be the result of an inner child wound being passed down your family line. Perhaps there's a version of how inner child wounds have been recycled in your family that's more specific to you. This could be a key opportunity to step back and reflect on what those intergenerational inner child transmissions have looked like and ask yourself the questions: (1) What was *modeled to* me? (2) What was *done to* me? and (3) What have I *never received*?

You will begin to find common threads when you start asking the same questions about your caregivers' childhoods and their caregivers' childhoods. The intergenerational commonalities and patterns start to become much more evident. These are often taken for granted because no one ever unpacked them. If not brought to light, they become normalized, and intergenerational. Learning to illuminate these wounds can be a first step in ensuring that you are not continuing to pass them on to your future generations. It's an initial step in the direction of you passing on emotional stability, safety, and maturity instead. These long-standing intergenerational childhood transmissions can end with you.

Emotionally Immature Parents

In a reasonably stable family, caregivers are able to be containers for the emotions of their children. They can tolerate a child's evolution, independence, rebellion, and needs. They encourage a healthy expression of all these emotions. However, in a family where harmful traits reside and emotional immaturity is the norm, an opportunity can remain open for intergenerational inner child wound transmissions. An emotionally immature caregiver is one who cannot adequately regulate their emotional triggers. Instead, they need others to manage their emotions for them. In some cases, those "others" are their children, because their children are vulnerable and accessible.

In families like this, children become the emotional depositories for their parents' unhealed pain. These parents may start to use their children for their own emotional support by oversharing with their children, producing what is called emotional incest, where children take on the role of an intimate partner with whom the parent can share all their worries and insecurities. This can lead children to internalize empathic stress. Empathetic stress is transmitted from parent to child as a result of the child observing their parent being overwhelmed and wishing to fix things for them. But most times, it's beyond a child's ability to cure their parent's pain. Instead, they continue to just ingest that pain and grow up to be adults who continue carrying that wound for their parents.

My client Leon's parents were emotionally immature. His mother, in particular, had a short fuse. This often led her to berate Leon verbally and physically. That is, unless she pushed Leon so far away that she then felt lonely, in which case she would use Leon's attention to fill the void. A common question she would ask Leon was "Do you love me?" This was often followed by "Do you think I'm a good mother?" And then by the grand finale of "Give your mother a hug." When she felt guilty for mistreating her child or when she felt her abandonment wound had been triggered, she would use her child to soothe her anguish. Leon was then taught that he needed to be the emotional blanket for his mother. She expected him to be her place of comfort. As a result, he long held on to the fantasy that he could save his mother from her pain. That he could heal the inner child that continued to hurt within her, so that she would no longer express her pain toward Leon. But stepping in to save a parent will leave the child with the inevitable consequence of neglecting their own needs, and in come those people-pleasing qualities. In order to disrupt this cycle of emotional immaturity, it's critical to learn how to self-soothe, heal your own inner child wounds, and attend to your attachment style.

Intergenerational Attachment Styles

Disruptions in your childhood will have an impact on the ways you connect to others. This is an undeniable fact. The quality of your connections to the people in your life will be contingent upon the quality of the connections you had in your formative years. When a child experiences healthy development, a parent who was able to work on their own inner child wounds, and one who was able to be emotionally mature, there's a solid base for learning a secure attachment style, meaning a safe and trusting connection to others. And secure attachments can offer a buffer against trauma. But when you don't have that foundation, or if the foundation is shaken at a critical point in your childhood, then it leaves room for emotional imbalance, followed by insecure attachments.

Remember the overactive intergenerational nervous system we learned about in chapter 6? Your caregiver's nervous system will either be settled and forge a connection with you or it will be overactive, which leaves little room for attunement. That poor attunement in childhood can then be the cause of ongoing attachment issues in adulthood. To establish security, both your physical and emotional needs need to have been met with consistency. This consistency allows both of your nervous systems to experience balance and attunement. Attachment theory proposes that a chronically stressed parent will not be likely to offer a secure attachment for their child. A nervous system that remains stuck in an unsafe place won't easily allow for a healthy connection, making it very hard, although not impossible, for a parent to form a secure attachment base for their children. A parent who struggles with rejection sensitivity and abandonment wounds and who can't emotionally connect with their child will find it hard to give their child what they themselves did not have.

As an adult, you may be prone to repeat the very dynamics of your childhood experience, and unconsciously enact the same attachment patterns with your own children. This is how a person can unwittingly become a cycle keeper. Or, you can opt to be a cycle breaker and choose the path of inner child healing, emotional maturity, and a secure attachment base. You can redirect the course of your lineage.

This was the decision that Leon made. He redirected the trajectory of these inner child transmissions when he had his own children. He became so intentional about reparenting himself and healing what generations in his family could not. As a result, he was able to disrupt a large part of those patterns as a parent. Just as Leon did, you can too. A first step for him, and now for you, was to capture how these patterns are showing up. This will require a deeper reflection, so pause and reflect on these questions to shed light into how the layers of attachment histories have made their way into your family life.

- Describe your relationship with your primary caretaker(s).
- What would happen when you needed them as a child (e.g., to provide love, nurturance, assistance, safety, etc.)?
- What types of emotions did it create in you to need them?
- In a few words, describe your caretaker's relationship with *their* caretaker(s).
- What would happen when they needed something as a child (e.g., help, love, nurturance, safety, etc.)?
- What emotions did it bring up for them to express a need for their own caretakers?
- Where are there similarities in the two attachment generations?
- Where are there differences in the two attachment generations?
- How would you like to disrupt the ways you attach with others, including the next generation, your descendants?

Healthy attachments are so critical for all of us. Humans are relational beings, which means that relationships will always be essential to our survival and well-being. So learning the layers of your attachment history and committing to establishing a different legacy will be a key aspect of how you function in your relationships from here forward. Let's take a moment to review how Yara managed to work through these childhood wounds to create her own legacy.

Yara's Abandonment Wound

My client Yara's father often failed to show up and take care of her. He was so inconsistent that Yara had a hard time trusting him, and one day when she was still fairly young, he forgot to pick her up from school. Yara felt abandoned, and her trust in her father's ability to care for her broke down. Then, Yara's mom and dad had a huge fight as a result, which led Yara to feel ashamed for needing her dad in the first place.

The fight was so enormous that Yara's father left that day and never returned. She murmured during our sessions, "If I hadn't needed him, this wouldn't have happened. He wouldn't have left."

For the rest of her childhood and into adulthood, she developed an intense self-sufficiency so that she could avoid the emotional load of abandonment. She never wanted to burden someone and carry the grief of them leaving ever again. But as she lightened the load for others, she placed an even bigger load on herself, the load of hyperindependence. She exhibited an overreliance on herself, led by the fear that others would let her down. And at the core of that hyperindependent behavior was a lack of trust in others. "I can't trust that others will show up for me" was the internal thought loop. Her life was organized around that fear. And if we were going to put the fragments back together, then we had to help Yara abandon that fear. We first dove into her intergenerational adverse experiences and started uncovering the layers. Her father had also been abandoned by one of his caregivers. This was an intergenerational wound, so Yara was even more determined to find her way out of the pattern.

Since Yara's abandonment wound was driven by the idea that she couldn't trust anyone to show up for her, our mission was to discredit that belief. So, we started with first helping her develop trust in small ways. We processed her discomfort with allowing someone to show up for her and worked on expanding her trust in the idea that she wasn't a burden. I told her, "You deserve the ease of trusting someone else, but let's start small and work our way up." Because Yara trusted my guidance, even if she still didn't trust herself or others, she believed in the value of the task. We were able to start that very day.

I asked Yara to make a simple request of a friend she had known for about five years. Their relationship wasn't very balanced, because thanks to her hyperindependence, Yara didn't allow this friend to do certain things for her. For example, over the years, her friend had more than once offered to pick Yara up when they would go out to concerts. But this was a huge trigger point for Yara, because it reminded her of that time when her dad didn't show up for her in school. This lack of trust had put some distance between Yara and her friend. So we set this small act of trust as our end goal: Yara would tolerate her friend picking her up for an event.

But we had to start small. At first, this meant allowing her friend to reserve their tickets. Then, it meant allowing her friend to pick up the concert tickets at will call for them. Each small moment of trust offered Yara an opportunity to reparent herself. Through this process, she learned what she needed to emotionally survive each next task. Sometimes the reparenting she offered herself was a deep breath. At other times, it was an affirmation that she wouldn't be abandoned again, and if so, that she could survive the experience.

Through this process, Yara started believing her father also needed reparenting, thanks to wounds from his own childhood. We had discussions about what it meant to know that he had also been abandoned by a caregiver. In sessions, we allowed some moments for processing how her own healing would be impacting her entire lineage, including her father. Yara was not forgiving or excusing her father for his abandonment, but simply acknowledging that her healing would have a generational impact. She was healing for herself and anyone else who couldn't. In time, Yara was able to disrupt those intergenerational child wounds and build trust with others. After months of building up to it, Yara was finally able to allow her friend to pick her up for an event that they attended together. But it all started with the trust she had in my ability to help her and the allowance she gave herself to sit in the discomfort of reparenting her own intergenerational inner child. An intergenerational reparenting process could do the same for you. It starts with breaking the cycles of parenting that haven't worked and shifting into a daily reparenting process that does. We will dive into what intergenerational reparenting can look like in the sections to come, but for now, let's take a deeper look at the parenting cycles that cycle breakers notice in their own healing journeys.

Breaking Parenting Cycles

Parenting is a skill that is mostly learned. Parents learn by observing other parents, including their own. And the reality is that if your grandparents were faulty in their parenting, that would have affected the ways your caregivers looked after you. Many times, parenting techniques are passed down from generation to generation. Harmful practices are oftentimes masqueraded as generational wisdom (e.g., "I have to hit you so you'll learn your lesson"). So many iterations of these harmful attitudes get handed down, become normalized, and then reproduce inner child wounds and insecure attachments. Some common yet harmful parenting beliefs and practices are:

- "I struggled, so you should struggle."
- "I never heard my mother tell me she loved me, and I turned out just fine."
- "I do it because I love you."
- "You'll thank me for this one day."
- "Children shouldn't put their nose in grown folks' business."
- "I can't go easy on you, because the world won't be easy on you."
- "You're the man/woman/person of the house now."
- "You need to learn right from wrong."
- "Children should be seen and not heard."
- "What I say goes and that's it."
- "But they're family."
- "You have to give them a hug and a kiss."
- "Cover up around men and boys."
- And so many others

And it isn't just the values that are translated into generational wounds. It's also the common sayings you heard growing up that can be internalized as harmful messages. It's the unkind and sometimes violent words that came out of your family members' mouths that stuck with you for life, such as:

- "I should've never had you."
- "Why can't you be more like your sibling?"
- "You're just like your father/mother."
- "Where did I go wrong with you?"
- "You were an accident."
- "Why can't you do anything right?"
- "I don't know what else to do with you."
- "You're too ugly/fat/thin/dark/gay."
- "If you weren't so difficult, we wouldn't be getting divorced."
- And so many others

It's also in the chronic invalidation that discounted your experiences and didn't allow you to naturally express your emotions, which also sent you a message about how you should process your emotions. Some examples of this include being told:

- "Suck it up."
- "Get over it already."
- "Stop being a wuss."
- "Man up."
- "It's not that big of a deal."
- "That's not really what happened."
- "You're so dramatic."
- "You don't actually feel that way."
- "You should be ashamed."
- "I don't believe you."
- "You're so lazy."

It's in the physical intrusion some children suffer that can contribute to their emotional arrest at the age of the physical violation. The pervasive lack of body boundaries that an adult can impose on you can leave you with scars that only you can see and feel. Others may not see them, but they are very much real and painful to you. These often include:

- Sexual molestation
- Hurting you physically
- A lack of body privacy, especially as you mature
- Having your body overly examined by way of Munchausen syndrome by proxy, which is when someone falsely claims that you have an illness in order to seek personal attention for themselves

It's in the things that were never given to you or the things that were taken away from you. And this can be either by way of the people in your family or by the systems that made it so that you suffered a disruption in care and affection. These include:

- Family members withholding love
- Receiving less affection than a sibling
- Not experiencing ongoing validation and affirmation
- Lack of attention to your basic needs (e.g., clean clothing, proper nutrition, etc.)
- Being placed in the foster care system and away from initial caretakers
- Being displaced by war, immigration, incarceration, or other systemic forces that took your caretakers' care away
- And any others that created a lack in your life

And it's in the feelings that these experiences left you with. Sometimes you don't have much recollection of how your family or an institution

caused you harm, because for some people, tragic childhoods become a
blur or a suppressed memory. But what you're left with is very telling of
the inequities of your childhood. And it can be found in the:

- Feeling of not being good enough
- Feeling like you have no control
- Feeling like you can't establish or sustain healthy boundaries
- Feeling an inner chaos, even when your life isn't externally chaotic
- Feeling like your needs are not to be taken seriously
- Feeling constantly misunderstood and not seen
- Feeling disregarded and not heard
- Feeling like you can't trust anyone
- Feeling like you can't trust yourself
- Feeling like you could never be loved
- Feeling like you have little power
- Feeling like you're perpetually broken

These behaviors and beliefs are learned in childhood. And the
teacher was almost always an adult in your life. These adults could have
been anyone who was close to you: grandparents, uncles, aunts, cousins,
siblings, religious institution members, neighbors, teachers, and prac-
tically any other community member with access to you or authority
over you who had an opportunity to injure you.

Caregivers tend to be the most common adults to cause this injury,
and it's a different type of hurt when it's a primary caregiver—after all,
they have an explicit duty to protect you. A caregiver is supposed to be
your default safe person. Yet still, whether it was a parent or community member, or whether that person hurt you consciously or unconsciously, that doesn't make a huge difference in how the hurt is
interpreted. Your young, developing mind registered the same message
either way. Regardless of who did the damage, the ultimate conse-

quences were the same: You became the adult with deep-seated inner child wounds, an emotional immaturity, or a fractured attachment style. You became the new bearer in a lineage of trauma. But just because that's the parenting legacy that came before you doesn't mean it's the legacy you have to pass along to the next generation. There are ways out of these patterns. And the way out starts with reparenting your intergenerational inner child. Now, let's do the work.

Breaking the Cycle: Intergenerational Reparenting

Reparenting is how you provide yourself with what you needed but didn't get as a child. It's how you help soothe your inner child and reconcile the wounds that have been there since you developed an emotional arrest. It is also the way in which you can repair insecure attachments and develop healthier relationships. This can be approached in a number of ways. Most notably, we start with reflections of what you needed as a child but didn't get, and then you start by offering yourself these reparenting moments in the present. They don't need to be in order. Simply practice what feels truest to your inner child's needs:

- Recite affirmations that you wish you heard as a child, such as "You are so lovable and worthy of that love."
- Give yourself a loving embrace that you missed having when you needed it.
- Offer yourself daily gifts of encouragement and love, like making yourself your favorite hot tea or buying yourself a soothing candle.
- Speak to yourself in a gentle, soothing tone.
- Re-create childhood memories, like watching a movie you loved back then.

- Engage in play, especially in playful activities that you missed in childhood, like playing on a swing at the park.
- Call up someone who offered you a sense of safety as a child or who does that for you now.
- Offer yourself opportunities to laugh out loud in a very childlike manner.
- And anything else that you specifically needed that was unique to your own childhood

And because here we are working through the layers of generations, reparenting also has to be intergenerational. That means that the work can also look like you helping your elders and ancestors reconcile the inner child wounds of their past. If someone is still living and you're willing to do this work with them, then you can invite them into the practice with you. If they are in the spirit world, you can journal to them about how you're also breaking this cycle on their behalf. If you need another, more tangible way to do this, I've got you. Just continue reading.

Grab a picture of yourself as a child, preferably at the age when you experienced emotional arrest.

- Look at that picture for 60 seconds and take in all the details.
- Breathe deeply, because this is likely the moment when your breathing is getting shallow.
- Remember that you are safe, you are here, you are an adult, and you are ready to give this child what they didn't receive in the past.
- If it helps, say those words out loud: "I am safe, I am here in the present, I am an adult, I am capable and ready to give my inner child what they need."
- Think back to the struggles of that time.
- Now, write down the ways in which your inner child struggled.

- Look at the picture and recite this mantra: "My sweet inner child, I release you from the pain of those who came before you, and I release you from the pain you suffered in this generation."
- To add the layers, reflect on the ways your inner child has been similar to the inner child of people whom you wish could also heal. These can be your parents, grandparents, siblings, or more distant ancestors.
- To further deepen the work, see if you can find pictures of living or past ancestors who you also wish to engage in an inner child affirmation exercise and recite the following: "My dear ancestor, I know your pain created an inner child wound in you too. I release that wound on your behalf and I will connect to my childlike joy for us both."
- Take many, many deep breaths.

This is a very mental and spiritual exercise, but I invite you to consider the ways your body is responding to this mantra. Pause and reflect on how offering yourself and your ancestors these liberatory affirmations has impacted you.

What You've Learned So Far

In this chapter, we explored how inner child traumas are passed down from generation to generation, and the relationship between trauma and attachment styles. You were guided through a number of intergenerational inner child wounds, the Intergenerational Adverse Experiences Questionnaire, and an intergenerational reparenting exercise. These concepts, as they are in real life, were intertwined, but also teased apart so you could grasp them a bit better, because the more you know, the more cycles you can disrupt. Once you're ready for some deeper reflections, transition to your reflection questions for this chapter and take a few deep breaths before diving into the next chapter, where we will get into cycles of abuse.

REFLECTION QUESTIONS

How was it for you to learn about the multiple layers of childhood adversity in your lineage?

What types of intergenerational inner child patterns were you able to identify in your family?

How was it for you to engage in the intergenerational reparenting exercise?

CHAPTER 8

Intergenerational Cycles of Abuse

Too many of us need to cling to the notion of love that either
makes abuse acceptable or at least makes it seem that
whatever happened was not that bad.

—bell hooks

Survivors of toxic abuse are often very psychologically attuned to others. That might be because they needed to be aware of minor changes in the emotions of the adults in their childhood environment for the sake of survival. In a home with an abusive or narcissistic parent, a sudden flash of anger can have violent consequences. When an emotionally vulnerable person, like a child, is exposed to abuse, they can consequently learn to continue repeating cycles of pain. If not challenged, the relationship patterns they were exposed to in their infancy can be the same dynamics they deem to be common and wind up cycling into later in life. Some of these dynamics can have a toxic quality and thus leave someone in a repetitive path of abuse. Let's continue ahead to learn about some common qualities of intergenerational abuse and the psychological remnants they can leave behind for generations.

Repeating Traumatizing Relationships

When chaos is all we know, chaos can feel familiar. An unfortunate reality for many traumatized people is that they will unconsciously continue repeating the same unhealthy behaviors and may have trouble learning how to break away from their repeated experiences. The hard-wired, subconscious drive that they have to repeat the familiar chaos is the basic premise of what is called *repetition compulsion*. It's when a person repeats a behavior over and over and reenacts old patterns time and again, even when they recognize that those patterns of behavior are harmful. Repetition compulsion manifests across all types of relationships: professional, romantic, with friends—all of them. It permeates a person's entire life.

This impulse becomes cyclical as each failed relationship confirms the negative beliefs you have deeply held (e.g., that people can't be trusted, that healthy relationships aren't possible, etc.). When these are the beliefs you have about yourself, others, and the world, you will repeat behaviors that reflect these internalized beliefs. I've seen this happen often with clients trying to break away from trauma. They are unconsciously driven to engage in a traumatic reenactment of past experiences in order to reconnect with the past, even if the past was deeply wounding. For example, they may rationalize when a partner mistreats them and continue to remain in toxic relationships. They can become enwrapped by a partner that displays the same relationship patterns they saw growing up. One such dynamic is codependency.

Codependency is a relationship pattern in which one person is constantly in need of another person's presence in order to help soothe their own emotions, even if the need is unconscious. Codependents enable each other and feed off each other in this cycle. In codependent relationships, people absorb each other's feelings, they feel a duty to fix each other's problems, and they become emotionally preoccupied with one another. Does that sound familiar? Children brought up in co-dependency can adopt those same relationship qualities as adults. It creates generational cycles of codependency and can cripple several family members' capacities to comfort themselves. It can also create a breeding ground for other unhealthy patterns of relationship dysfunction and abuse. Although these cycles produce negative consequences, they can be emotionally rewarding to go back to because they feel so familiar. Because they feel like home.

As a cycle breaker, however, you don't want to be stuck in these patterns anymore. Instead, you want past wounds to heal. You don't want to find yourself repeating those harmful cycles. You want to break free from them. The good news is that with the proper knowledge and strategy, you can stop reenacting the past and adversely impacting your current relationships. You can learn new strategies for breaking these intergenerational abuse cycles.

How Cycles of Abuse Continue

More often than not, relationships that start with power, manipulation, codependency, or other toxic habits end that way. They follow a certain pattern. This pattern is the cycle of abuse. A cycle of abuse, which is also referred to as a cycle of violence, describes a pattern of behaviors used to gain or maintain power and control over another person in a relationship, and is typically characterized by a power imbalance. Generally, one person uses abusive behaviors to control the other person. At their worst, these behaviors can be terrifying, leading to life-threatening or even fatal acts of violence.

Children who suffered in these cycles of abuse are at a greater risk of perpetuating the same cycles in their adult intimate relationships. Since this has been modeled to them, it can become what they reenact in their adult lives. But a conscious understanding of what these patterns are can act as a buffer against repeating them. In order to avoid violent, dysfunctional, and abusive relationships, key stages of this cycle need to be identified. The four stages of abuse are:

- **The Tension-Building Stage**—this is where the perpetrator of toxic dynamics starts showing signs of frustration and building tension in the relationship. The person on the receiving end of the toxic behavior will likely be trying to appease the other person to avoid a blowup.
- **The Incident Stage**—this is where there's an eruption of the tension, and controlling behavior takes center stage. Typically, this involves threats, humiliation, gaslighting (manipulating someone into questioning their own sanity or rendition of events), and isolation.
- **The Reconciliation Stage**—this stage is also called the "honeymoon" phase, and is where the perpetrator tries to reestablish a connection, likely shows remorse, bombs the person with love gestures (this is called *love bombing*, or the act of overwhelming a person with over-the-top, insincere gestures and promises of love), and makes a commitment to not continue the undesired behavior, typically with the end goal of gaining back trust. Many times that accountability doesn't happen, and instead they will gaslight their victim so that they will be the one to apologize and believe the abuse was their fault.
- **The Calm Stage**—this is where things are fairly peaceful but eventually gearing up toward building tension again. Here you are feeling a false sense of calm. You are bracing yourself to experience another tension-building phase.

These traumatic ups and downs can counterintuitively make relationships feel stronger, also known as *trauma bonding*. And it's how the people in these relationships keep each other unwell. Breaking free of these types of cycles will require difficult, layered work. Yet at the center of that liberation is how you create a new identity that has balance, not chaos and toxic abuse, at the center.

Toxic Abuse

In order to understand the mistreatment of others, we have to dive into the personality characteristics that contribute to it. Recognizing toxic traits is important in breaking cycles, because being in a close familial, friendly, or romantic relationship with a person who has harmful qualities can be traumatic and produce generations of pain. This type of experience can be at the center of your trauma responses and can inhibit you from being your truest, highest intergenerational self. In the worst case, you might absorb these traumatic behaviors and unwittingly pass them along to the people in your life and to the next generation. So, identifying these toxic traits is actually a tool for cycle breaking, because it teaches you to recognize abusive personality characteristics that have the ability to cause deep, intergenerational trauma.

Some toxic people have malicious intent. Others might just lack the capacity and tools to engage in healthier relationship dynamics, even if they desire to. Regardless of whether toxic action is deliberate, conscious, or unconscious, it isn't excusable and it can be *terrorizing to the person that's targeted*. People with toxic tendencies might know how to disarm you. They can weaponize their understanding of your vulnerabilities and use them to control you. They can drain you in their efforts to cater to their own needs.

I once had a client, Solomon, whose boyfriend would smile with deep pleasure to know that he had caused my client pain. His partner locked my client's cat out of the house for weeks after the cat destroyed their furniture. He would ask my client, "What are you going to do about it?" while standing over him in order to intimidate him and leverage his power over my client. Then he would yell, "You're going to do nothing. Now go make yourself useful before I throw you out with that dirty cat of yours." As a result, Solomon would shrink and squirm in fear. My client was being controlled, a victim of his partner's toxic abuse. As time went on, his partner became increasingly violent, his abuse escalating. He would oftentimes lock the door to the apartment, leaving my client outside for the night. On those nights, his partner would sleep serenely while Solomon was left to cry himself to sleep outside their front door. His partner dozed off with no empathy, regard, or remorse for Solomon's feelings or safety. This is a characteristic of a deliberate pathological toxicity that is severe and damaging to others, to the point where healing from these damaging effects in one generation can be hard, although not impossible. It has taken my client a long time to recover from the effects of this relationship. It has taken even longer for him to notice the stark similarities between these toxic dynamics and the ones he saw growing up. Opening his eyes to both generations of toxicity was a part of the damage control we needed to engage in. It all began with my client's conscious understanding of toxic abuse cycles and the ways in which he was stuck in the cycles he saw growing up.

A close relationship with a toxic person can tear through your life like a tornado. If you've been through this, you know what I mean. It hurts. Deeply. So deep you feel like you'll never recover. I'm here to tell you that you can, with work and the tools I offer here, but it's understandable if it feels like a big task. In my professional experience, I've found that the best armor against harmful behaviors is knowledge. I can't stress enough how empowered my clients feel when they find themselves capable of identifying something that's been hurtful for ages and finally speaking up. For example, having the knowledge to say, "That's gaslighting," to someone who is attempting to distort your sense of reality can be such a great source of empowerment—vastly different from sitting in the confusion of being gaslighted. With that power, you can develop an added guard against toxic behaviors, because you now understand what toxic traits actually are. I'd like to take some time to help you disarm toxic behaviors—perhaps toxic behaviors you have been the victim of, or perhaps toxic behaviors that you yourself have been displaying—by knowing more about them.

Examples of some toxic traits include:

- Manipulating others to supply one's own needs
- Engaging in controlling behavior to restrict others from contacting friends or family
- Limiting resources, like money
- Engaging in highly negative and pessimistic behaviors that cause others to feel chronically invalidated
- Being physically intrusive to someone in a way that violates them physically
- Being sexually intrusive to someone in a way that violates them sexually
- Lying chronically and perpetuating dishonesty
- Exhibiting cruel and spiteful behavior
- Treating people as possessions and engaging in jealous behavior when that person can't be controlled
- Claiming no responsibility or accountability but instead making a habit of blaming others
- Gaslighting others in order to twist reality to manipulate the narrative of what happened
- Casting constant judgment on others and believing themselves to be a fair judge of other people's actions
- Making a conscious effort to create chaos

Get to know this list. Reflect on it. And equip yourself with a healthy emotional guard against people who display these traits. This is a part of how you protect yourself and your lineage from the unhealthy effects of toxicity. This is how you start the process of breaking these cycles, through the knowledge of how they manifest and continue. And if you read some of these and thought, "Welp, that sounds just like me," I'm glad you're growing in your awareness and are willing to do the work to put an end to the toxic traits you've adopted throughout your life. This isn't meant to cause you shame but to increase your knowledge about how you can also replicate hurt in others. This is also not meant to condone any of your harmful behaviors, because it is your responsibility to change them. You have to make a conscious choice to break free from the destructive patterns you have held on to. You committing to change is necessary. Not just for you but also for the people who need you to no longer hurt them.

Recycling Abuse

My client Nola lived in perpetual misery. She carried that misery all her life. She never felt safe, integrated, or joyous, because she came from a family and a place where toxicity ran rampant. She lived in a house in the southern United States with both her mother and father for most of her childhood, but she sometimes felt like she lived with no parents at all. She was the eldest of five siblings, a parentified child who took care of the younger four, and a child of parents who were both living with addictions. One parent was addicted to alcohol while the other was addicted to gambling. Both parents would use up their family funds on their respective addictions and would later be infuriated when the family didn't have enough money to cover their basic needs. Her parents would engage in rageful and violent attacks against each other and toward their children to unload their desperation for more money.

Nola's parents came from a long line of people who had lived with addiction and domestic violence. How they behaved in their relation-ship mirrored what they had witnessed in their own childhood homes. Accordingly, these became the default behaviors they modeled to Nola and her siblings. As a kid, Nola would try to resolve their fights, but she felt defeated by the realization that she couldn't help them, despite all her efforts. Eventually she stopped trying, but she never stopped hurt-ing. Nola developed deep, complex intergenerational trauma, marked by the toxic abuse she experienced.

When we started working together, Nola was having a lot of trouble adjusting to her new job as a social worker and felt that her supervisor tended to create more work for her than was necessary. In session with me, she would call her supervisor an "absolute idiot." She complained about how her boss made her job "so much harder than it needed to be" and how she would have to spend time and energy fixing her boss's er-rors. This would be a frustrating problem to have, sure. But I was more interested in understanding why these experiences with her supervisor had the power to spiral Nola to the point of a depression. And then why, in her depression, she would become irritable, impatient, and downright cruel toward people at work.

"This feels deeper than what you're describing, Nola," I would say to her. "Here you are, needing to fix people's problems that they should be able to fix themselves, in the same ways that you felt you had to fix your parents' problems as a child." Her childhood frustrations of having two parents who couldn't fix their own issues were coming back up with her supervisor's inability to do the same. I was aiming to show her the intergenerational triggers that were surfacing, to help her understand why her intergenerational nervous system was entering fight mode in her everyday life. If she stayed angry, she wouldn't have to confront the deeper sorrow she felt when people, anyone, let her down. She wouldn't have to face the grief she carried over having parents who couldn't break the cycle. Her anger was her defense against the deep despair she held.

In her moments of cruelty against others, she felt deep shame. She hated how triggered she became when people let her down. It was causing her pain, but she didn't know why, and she didn't know how to address it. A part of the solution was to help her process the toxic stress she had endured and learn how to cope with stress triggers better so that she wouldn't perpetuate suffering for others.

In psychology, we have a set of practices that help a person increase their ability to manage emotional distress. If you have a history of stress and trauma, chances are that you will have a low tolerance for stress, meaning that any mild stressor could overwhelm you and land you back in harmful cycles. Learning how to tolerate stress better can help you decrease emotional overwhelm in your life and manage your emotions in a way that feels healthier and more productive, rather than destructive, painful, and toxic. I developed a practice called STILL that is geared toward increasing stress tolerance. My clients and I use it to process the strain of the past and the stress of the present. Let's learn more about this skill below.

Breaking the Cycle: Increasing Your Capacity to Tolerate Stress with STILL

Greater mindfulness of your emotions offers you a widened capacity to feel your feelings without acting on them. Once you're able to tolerate the stress that's inside your body, welcome it, and understand what it's trying to tell you, and once you're able to feel your feelings and resist the urge to immediately act on them, then you will have gained a new and highly effective skill in better managing your emotions. This is powerful cycle-breaking behavior. Importantly, I'd like for you to practice this skill when you're *not* feeling deeply fired up. It's critical for you to be able to practice with mildly stressful situations first. This way, you can build up the skill while in a calmer state, so you develop a greater chance of making it more of a default when you need it in times of high stress.

I call this practice STILL, which stands for Stop, Temperature, Inhale, Lay, Launch. This skill gives you an opportunity to quickly shift to cooling your body down and rerouting your mind so that you don't act on the explosive emotions that are getting ready to surface. The more you can exert healthy control over yourself, the more you can influence how you express your emotions to other people. Here are the steps:

- **Stop**—Picture a stop sign in your mind. This will remind you to freeze in place and not do anything rash that can jeopardize your well-being or relationships. It helps if you remove yourself from the situation as completely as possible.
- **Temperature**—Grab an ice pack and hold it in your hands, splash your face with cold water, go outside and feel the brisk air on your skin, or dip your body in cold water. The cold temperature helps your body create endorphins, which are hormones that help your nervous system feel less stressed. It's the physical version of cooling off your emotions.
- **Inhale**—You are continuing to engage your nervous system to reestablish a sense of calm in your body. Breathe in for 5 seconds and out for 7 seconds each time. Do this for no less than 5 minutes, since your nervous system needs at least that amount of time to create a parasympathetic relaxation response that helps you feel calmer.
- **Lay**—Pause and lie down for a few minutes to take a break from the situation and gather your thoughts about it. If possible, I would suggest even sitting and rocking yourself to increase the relaxation response of your ventral vagal nerve.

- **Launch**—Your next course of action should come from a more regulated state, so feel free to now move forward with the situation, since you won't be doing so from an elevated emotional state but from a calmer one. Now you can head back into the conversation with a more regulated nervous system.

Repeat this sequence as often as you need to. The more you repeat it, the greater your emotion regulation. The greater your regulation, the more that you'll behave from a place that elicits pride instead of shame. The more that you follow that pattern, the more you'll disrupt the other patterns that were previously concretized in your mind and body. The more that you disrupt older patterns, the more that you'll be able to adopt a personality that is centered on stillness, rather than chaos.

What You've Learned So Far

In this chapter, you learned about the ways in which intergenerational cycles of abuse perpetuate intergenerational trauma. Within those cycles, we have certain personality characteristics that can be toxic and create deep wounds in you and in your family. Because knowledge helps you exercise more power, you learned about these characteristics and cycles in depth. You also learned an important mechanism for helping you through toxic stress, the STILL technique. This chapter may have brought up some heavy memories, but I also hope it has empowered you with helpful knowledge to build up your intergenerational healing toolbox. If you're hoping for more tools, keep reading through your reflection questions below and head over to the next chapter, where we'll be covering how collective trauma makes its way into your home and family.

REFLECTION QUESTIONS

How was it to learn about the ways in which you may be engaging in
intergenerational cycles of abuse?

What came up for you as you read through the list of toxic traits?

How do you feel about practicing STILL on a daily basis to increase
your stress tolerance?

CHAPTER 9

When Collective Trauma Enters
Your Home

We have to talk about liberating minds as well as liberating
society.

—Angela Davis

Understanding intergenerational trauma healing requires that we not just look closely into your family dynamics but that we also dig into the external factors that bring intergenerational trauma into your home in the first place. We each have relationships with people, institutions, and the larger world. Each of these has some influence over our lives. So, when looking at intergenerational trauma, it is critical to zoom out and see the other factors that also contribute to keeping these cycles going.

None of us live in silos, but rather within an entire ecosystem with different moving parts. Our families are a part of that ecosystem, and they are influenced by cultures that maintain a specific set of values that keep these cycles going. Within that same ecosystem, we also have the institutions and systemic structures with the power, and indeed the propensity, to breed harmful norms and practices that then perpetuate trauma. And then there's the larger world, which spans beyond our person-made cultural or institutional control, but can also have the ability to incapacitate our families via trauma. All of these— the cultural influences, the systemic influences, and the natural world influences—are added culprits of intergenerational trauma. If we are to disrupt cycles at the root, then we have to take inventory of what's feeding those roots: collective trauma.

The Wounds of Collective Trauma

Collective trauma is the experience of extreme adversity of a group of people. This type of trauma creates a collective memory, a remembrance of something that has been deeply damaging to the spirit of a community. It is the consequence of harmful cultural values (e.g., the belief that children are to be seen and not heard, the belief that people can just get over their depression, etc.), systemic oppression of a group of people (e.g., economic suppression, racial oppression, sexism, heterosexism, etc.), and natural disasters (e.g., earthquakes, hurricanes, pandemics, etc.). Emotional injury that is caused at a collective level creates psychological reactions, many of which mirror the symptoms that happen at the individual and family level. It has been found that collective traumas can lead to both immediate and lifelong mental health conditions such as depression, anxiety, and post-traumatic stress disorder. Descendants of trauma sufferers have been found to absorb an intergenerational transmission of shock, meaning that they take on the shock of those who suffered the original trauma.

Through several points of research, we have seen the secondary trauma found down the lineage of descendants of African chattel slavery and racial caste systems, Aboriginal descendants of massacres and land dispossession, Native descendants of colonial terror and genocide, Middle Eastern descendants of war and the cultural complexities of displacement, South Asian descendants of partitions and exclusions,

East Asian descendants of refugees and the disenfranchisement that's experienced as a result, descendants of Holocaust survivors, and so many other collectives of people. Psychological impacts have also been found in descendants of natural disasters across the world. Some of these larger-scale circumstances can also cause a disruption to the soul, because they are a part of the vast web of intergenerational trauma. There's a layered connection between collective and individual traumas, because a lot of what happens in the home has external roots. These larger-scale issues seep into the crevices of our homes and cause wounds that can remain unresolved for generations.

As you read, you may already be considering some external influences that are a part of how intergenerational trauma has been maintained in your family. That's important. This is a moment in which you can get curious about these external factors. You may find that thinking about the enormous impact of external influences can even make you feel like you have little control to change them. It can feel like the imposition of trauma on your soul won't end in your generation, or even in several generations to come. But that couldn't be further from the truth. Cycle breakers, like you, change family, community, and societal dynamics on a larger scale every day. You can create a shift that, no matter how small, can impact many generations into the future. So hold your heart steady as you read another piece of this intergenerational web and know that you *can* also do something about this external layer. If it helps, pause here and take a few deep breaths. With each breath, recite the mantra in your mind "I can create change. And the change I create matters." And take a final breath before diving back in. As you already know, we cannot change what we cannot see, so it will be critical to gather a more comprehensive understanding of how each of these layers of collective trauma (the cultural, the systemic, and the natural) can create or influence intergenerational trauma in you and others.

What Happened Around You?

Remember the modified Intergenerational Adverse Experiences Questionnaire that Leon and I started? When we began to explore the portion of the questionnaire that asks "What happened around you? (Community or Societal Collective Adversity)," Leon and I were able to uncover a host of different collective traumas that were a part of his story. Physical abuse was normalized in his community (check); his ancestors were victimized by the chattel slavery imposed upon and subsequent institutionalized oppression of Black Americans (check); his family had to evacuate their home due to Hurricane Katrina (check). I felt like the checks just kept coming. One person, one mind, one body, one spirit, and one complicated living collective history. For Leon, this was a part of his intergenerational history that could not be left behind. Collective trauma was also a part of his life at the cultural level, through the multigenerational influences in his family that made it culturally acceptable for his parents to use physical violence as a child-rearing practice. Collective trauma was also present in his life through systemic trauma and the historical trauma he suffered from the legacies of oppression of people of the African diaspora. He was also contending with the collective trauma of Hurricane Katrina, which he had survived physically, but by which he had been scarred mentally and spiritually.

Many of us who bear intergenerational trauma check several boxes on the modified ACES questionnaire. And cycle breakers, like yourself, tend to want to reflect on their own experiences of collective traumas and understand the ways in which these have also been implicated in their generational pain. To get you started, think back to the "What Happened Around You?" portion of the questionnaire we worked through in chapter 7. But this time, consider the three layers of collective trauma and how each has had an influence in your life. Then continue reading to gather a wider understanding of each level of collective trauma.

Cultural Influences

Our families are embedded in a complex web of cultural values. There is no doubt that we become an embodiment of the values we grew up with in our families and communities. These values and practices have formed over generations and thus are deeply ingrained in our community identities. Take, for example, the act of physically punishing a child as a child-rearing practice. In many cultures around the world, and for many generations, physical abuse of children has been considered to be an acceptable parenting practice. In the Black community in America, some have used a switch to forcibly change a child's behavior. In the Latine culture, there's also a common symbol of physical beatings, *la chancla*, or the slipper, the tool used to force children into submission. Even the mere raising of a chancla, without it being used to inflict pain, is sufficient for Latine children to understand that they need to listen to their parent's request. Some Latine cultures have also been known to resort to more painful items as disciplinary tools, like tree branches.

Various cultures have a version of the switch, branches, and la chancla. Some use belts, and others use anything they can find that will inflict physical pain to control children's behavior. Working with families, but also being a Black Latina myself, I've seen it all. The object may be different, but the impact is the same. These are tools of power that inflict fear. Children who are exposed to this kind of terror will seek to avoid the pain by succumbing to their caregiver's request. And their caregiver will see that changed behavior and be reinforced to believe that the strategy of hitting their child actually worked. Although this may temporarily be the case, what is simultaneously taking place is that their child's nervous system is being programmed around fear and fear-avoidance. So, while their child effectively avoided a temporary state of terror by changing their behavior, they also assumed a more long-term coping method of pleasing others to avoid experiencing fear. Unfortunately, many children who suffer this fate will have their nervous system rewired to be frozen in a default sympathetic state, meaning that they will have an overactive threat alert system that keeps them in prolonged states of panic well into their adulthood.

If we dig deeper into history, particularly the historical trauma of colonization across the world, physical punishment was a major tool used to instigate submission and fear. In many of the cultural practices that followed, physical abuse became indoctrinated, passed on as a cultural value, and replicated, generation after generation, in home after home, until it reached you. These practices have roots in colonization yet have remained etched in family histories that contribute to daily present-day occurrences of intergenerational traumas. When you crafted your Intergenerational Trauma Tree, you were prompted to add to the soil some of the cultural norms and practices that were feeding the roots (your ingrained beliefs). These are likely the cultural beliefs that are most prominently reflected in your intergenerational trauma journey. However, this moment offers another healthy pause to consider additional examples of what other cultural beliefs have been floating through your communities that have fed those roots. Other examples of how cultural values get translated into lasting emotional trauma are the following (this is not an exhaustive list, just one to help you get curious about your own cultural values):

- Believing that an elder child (usually eldest daughter) should care for their younger siblings, known as parentification, which can strip them of their childhood and produce inner child wounds and emotional suppression that then get replicated for generations

- Telling young girls to cover up to avoid the attention of men, which can send multiple messages about the objectification of their bodies, which they then pass on as added gendered cultural values to their daughters
- Believing that a child must always be kind to elders, even the elders who hurt them, which can lead them to suppress their own feelings and to people-pleasing tendencies that they then teach their own kids
- Believing that secrets must be kept in the family, otherwise you destroy honor, which can lead a person to self-isolate or not seek help when feeling stressed; instead of resolving any trauma that's absorbed, they risk passing it on
- Protecting perpetrators of childhood molestation at the expense of the children they hurt, which can dissuade a person from speaking up about being violated and can keep perpetrators assailing children for lack of accountability
- Bleaching skin practices that perpetuate the systemized belief that darker skin is undesirable, which leads children to absorb these soul-destroying messages that can lead to adverse health consequences that get transmitted generationally, together with the transmission of low self-esteem
- Commenting on the weight and appearance of children in order to fit ill-informed societal standards, which can contribute to body image issues and eating disorders, which are then modeled to subsequent generations
- Passing on the idea that boys don't cry, which can contribute to an oversuppression of emotions in boys and men, which can then underwrite generations of toxic masculinity
- And many, many, many others

Because these major cultural factors can feel so close to home, they can be hard to tease out and examine in the bigger picture. So it can help to sit and write a list of how your cultures have influenced your thinking. From there, you can identify positive influences (e.g., helping you keep a healthy sense of identity, helping you learn the value of maintaining harmony in your family and community, etc.) versus influences that can cause harm. Once you're done with that step, start considering the ways in which you are already disrupting the collective influence you've internalized. For example, if you are a part of a culture where it has been normalized to punish children through physical violence, you might choose to break the cycle by not hitting your own children but also by helping other parents in your family (e.g., your cousins or siblings) find gentle, nonphysical methods of discipline. This can help settle your own intergenerational nervous systems, rather than further traumatize your children.

Breaking the cycle in these ways (by helping yourself and assisting others whom you can easily reach) can be helpful and empowering when considering the enormity of these cultural issues. Something I find to be helpful is to envision myself approaching the issue and dismantling it. So often we feel like the issue is so large that it can overtake us, but when we visualize the issue as more approachable and less overburdening, it can help us feel less tentative about taking action. Take a few deep breaths as you think about these some more, before moving into the ways systemic factors function as a driver of collective traumas.

Systemic Influences

Like cultural influences, systemic factors can remain hidden for generations. Typically, what hides them are a set of uncontested institutional practices that have been considered standard or the norm.

Have you ever heard of septic shock? It's when an infection becomes widespread and starts causing organ failure across the entire body. It's a gruesome full-system meltdown caused by untreated bacteria. Systemic injustice can have a similar effect culturally. Untreated, it will infect everything. A system of oppression is one that is intended to hurt and damage the life of certain targeted groups while elevating and privileging others. In the US, but also across the world, we have many systems intentionally diseased in this way that were built to oppress, persecute, mistreat, tyrannize, enslave, imprison, exploit, occupy, and afflict chronic mental, physical, and spiritual pain upon marginalized communities. I call these *diseased systems*, because they're contaminated with harm. Many have been built with the explicit aim of doing harm and are masterful in carrying out that mission. These systems cause and perpetuate collective trauma daily and infect entire groups and communities through the mechanism of institutional power and control.

Those who fall prey to these diseased systems develop distress at insurmountable levels. A commonplace example of this can be found in the experience of *post-traumatic slave syndrome*, the consequence of the multigenerational oppression of Africans and their descendants as a result of centuries of chattel slavery and institutionalized racism. The term was developed by Dr. Joy DeGruy to help answer the question "What happens when stressed people lack treatment for generations?" Because institutionalized racism of Black people across the Americas has never ceased, the legacy of post-traumatic slave syndrome—one marked by collective hypervigilance, mistrust, hopelessness, and a distorted self-concept—persists. It is a collective trauma that continues to be recycled through the generations.

Other examples of how systemic norms and practices get translated into emotional trauma are the following (this is not an exhaustive list, just one to help you get curious about your own connections):

- Educational systems that have exceptionally punitive disciplinary practices toward Black, Indigenous, and people of color (BIPOC) and are the initial point of the criminalization of BIPOC youth and the subsequent funneling into the criminal injustice system, which leads to the separation of families and multigenerational economic depravity

- Social systems that privilege one population over another and place higher value on one collective of humans over another, leading to intergenerational internalization of lack of worthiness, lack of belonging, perceived inferiority, impostor syndrome, low self-esteem, collective self-esteem, and *so* much more
- Wars that displace families, who then seek refuge and asylum elsewhere, only to be confronted with a different set of institutional traumas and the children who subsequently absorb the immigrant and refugee traumas of their parents as a result
- Forced assimilation into dominant cultures at the expense of lost cultures, languages, and traditions of land natives, which can lead to a disruption in a community's identity and self-concept, and the collective soul of an entire population
- The financial institutions that keep the already marginalized intergenerationally poor and demolish their access to tools that can help them build social mobility, which contributes to multigenerational poverty trauma
- The societal assumptions around who people should love or how they should self-identify, which causes identity-based traumas and can be the setup for the transmission of stress-based biologies
- The laws that impose patriarchal rules on the bodies of anyone with a uterus and place great danger on their bodies, which can lead to pregnancy, postpartum, or uterine health complications, or even death
- The systems that tyrannize or discredit various religious and spiritual beliefs in the service of one dominant belief system and that allow for the victimization of people who don't subscribe to dominant beliefs, who then suffer religious traumas as a result
- The health-care systems that exploit the bodies of BIPOC, sometimes even killing people in the name of so-called science,

like the murders enacted during the unethical Tuskegee Study of
Untreated Syphilis, where African American men were injected
with syphilis and not offered education or treatment of the
disease, often leading to death and to a multigenerational cultural
mistrust of the health-care system, which further perpetuates the
intergenerational health disparities that disproportionately impact
Black people in the US

- And many, many, many others

The experience of post-traumatic slave syndrome also offers an example of how much Black individuals continue to fight and persist
through generational resilience by maintaining cultural language, histories, and values that keep the collective esteem of the community
alive and thriving, despite multigenerational oppression and terror.
Regardless of the ongoing disruptions to the Black soul, produced by
the diseased society that Black people exist in, an immense amount of
resilience and cultural pride burgeon from the souls of Black people
every day. Similar expressions of multigenerational resilience can be
found in other communities that have been victimized by diseased systems. So when thinking about your own experiences, especially chronic
ones like this, it can be helpful to also consider how you have survived
and thrived, despite being in a world that doesn't desire that for you.

Systemic norms and practices can take time to understand and de-
construct. One thing you can do right now, however, is to consider
how systemic inequities pour into your life in ways that feel stressful or
traumatizing. How have you been impacted by these systems? Take a
moment to pause and reflect on the ways they may have perpetuated
trauma for you and your family. And as with the cultural values reflection, it can also help here to consider the things you could do in order
to combat systems that oppress you and others in these traumatic ways.

One way I have seen my parents fight the injustices perpetuated on economically deprived immigrant populations is by going into their local community and helping boost the Latine vote during elections. As working-class immigrants themselves, they understood that bringing our voices to the ballot was an effective way to help protect our families from the inequities of immigration laws, which caused my family to suffer from a ten-year separation. I decided to use my practice of holistic trauma healing to provide sound bath meditations for my community during the wave of heavy collective crisis and collective grief that we as a world experienced in 2020. These practices may not be easy, but acting within our power is a necessary part of the web of creating equality and healing in our communities. We can each do something that helps.

What are some accessible ways you could fight to diminish systemic trauma in your communities? I find that it can be helpful to start small, then scale up. These issues will take time to undo, but a tiny act can go a long way. And although it is not the sole responsibility of those who have been wounded systemically to dismantle these systems, if you have been victimized by these systems, your efforts also matter and can bring you a sense of empowerment, especially given how you have been incessantly rendered to exist with diminished power. If you are privileged by these systems, you have an even greater duty to disrupt them and their impact, given the power and access that you hold to do so. And if you are having trouble seeing how you are explicitly either privileged or disenfranchised by these systems and their ideologies, your unfamiliarity should motivate you to expand your consciousness and shift into action. Rest assured that if, as a result of your lack of awareness, you choose the path of neutrality and inaction, your lack of effort to disrupt will not save you from being infected by that system's harmful ideas and practices. So what's one thing that you can do now? Once you reflect and write, be sure to breathe before diving into the more natural forces that can also harm us generationally.

Natural Influences

People can also develop vulnerabilities due to traumas driven by natural forces. For some, hidden traumas may surface, while for others,
added traumas get layered on top of what they were already dealing
with. The COVID-19 pandemic, for example, triggered a whopping 25
percent increase in depression, anxiety, addictions, and suicidal ideation worldwide. The widespread fear, loss, and trauma were deeply felt
within every generation, in every home across the world. People lost
jobs, parents, children, a sense of safety, and so much more. That prolonged trauma shock is an example of a modern-day natural disaster
and its impact on our entire families.

For any of us, recovering from a natural crisis can be a lengthy process, typically taking over a decade for significant resolution to occur.
This is especially so if we suffered a loss during that time, like many did
during the COVID-19 pandemic. If your nervous system was already
vulnerable, it will take even longer to feel at ease. This is typical. It is
expected. We need time to recover from acute periods of stress. Recovery is possible, but it takes patience and collective effort. As a person
who experienced this pandemic, you can reflect on the ways in which
multiple generations of your family have been directly impacted by this
collective crisis and other natural crises. It is said that young people
have especially felt the burden of the ongoing natural crises that they
continue to witness. The US Surgeon General, Dr. Vivek Murthy,
noted in a talk with Oprah Winfrey on the UCLA Health campus in
May 2023 that mental health is the "defining public health crisis of our
time." Additionally, he noted in an interview with the *New York Times*
that for young Americans in particular, the stress of compounded natural disasters is one of the notable reasons for their mental health de-
cline, since these continuous disasters have negatively impacted their
perceptions of the future. The effects of these ongoing natural crises are

concerning for many, across generations, so if you share these concerns, know that it is understandable to feel this way and that it is essential to pause and check in with yourself and others.

If you choose to pause here and write some reflections, remember to take deep breaths, because the impact of this pandemic is very recent and can cause your breath to shorten as you reflect. If it helps, start with writing some answers to the following: What prominent emotion did you feel during the height of the pandemic? How was your body carrying the weight of the pandemic? What relationship disruptions happened during this period? Once you've reflected, it can be healthy to go back into breathing deeply a few more times before returning to reading. When you're ready, continue reading to learn how these natural traumas make their way into our homes.

The following examples represent how natural disasters can translate to emotional trauma (this is not an exhaustive list, just one to help you reflect on the impact of this external factor):

- The powerful destruction of Hurricane Katrina in New Orleans, which was followed by a lack of efficient and prompt relief by government bodies, which then left entire families in water for days, swimming in deplorable conditions, and with smell and trauma imprints of death and defecation to last generations, among other harmful consequences
- The ongoing wildfires in the western regions of the continental United States and on Maui, which destroyed homes and businesses and promptly displaced families from their homes as a result, and which will leave a multigenerational impact of loss and grief
- The compounded destruction of villages in Haiti due to earthquakes and the lack of expedient rebuilding of infrastructures across the land, which have led many families to experience homelessness and even more profound poverty trauma that will impact the nation's people for generations

- The Tohoku earthquake and tsunami that killed over 15,000 people and displaced another 450,000 others and crippled the infrastructure of the entire country of Japan, leaving trauma memories in multiple generations of Japanese people and their descendants
- The ongoing floods in Nigeria that have impacted a total of 1.5 million people, which have led to community displacements, loss of businesses, loss of homes, and loss of life, which will require many generations of both psychological and logistical rebuilding

When Hurricane Maria devastated millions of lives in Puerto Rico, Dominica, and Saint Croix, the islands were in need of relief efforts from the entire worldwide community, and for many, help didn't come in time or at all. I remember the tears of devastation from my Puerto Rican client who felt newly disempowered by this crisis in Puerto Rico, where some of her family members still resided. She took to activism work around climate change to help corporations increase climate responsibility as a way to feel empowered to help her community for generations to come. Another client's family was evacuated due to a typhoon in the Philippines in late 2021, which was compounded by the COVID-19 pandemic still impacting the region. She decided to initiate a funding campaign in order to help the disaster relief efforts in her local community. Both felt that this was a collective trauma they wanted to fight, for themselves and the future descendants of their communities. Your devotion to natural relief efforts could look different from either of these. However, if natural crises have been in your history, and if you feel motivated to help, this can be a place to find a sense of empowerment, community, and healing.

If It Feels Like Too Big of a Task

Remember that one small change, by any one of us, is compounded with the efforts of others. Eventually, our collective efforts lead to tangible changes that we can see in our generation. And if you're ever feeling stuck, be mindful of some of the major internal messages that can keep us in inaction:

- Believing that collective trauma is too big for us to tackle
- Believing that our ancestors are not here to help us
- Believing that we have to solve it all in one shot
- Believing that once a collective trauma has passed, it won't come back to impact us emotionally, spiritually, physically, culturally, or structurally
- Believing that we are not complicit in the continuation of collective traumas (especially anyone who upholds the values of a toxic system, even if they themselves are the people whom the system oppresses)
- Believing in the superiority of one group of people over another
- Believing that a sense of power and privilege will keep us safe
- Believing that intergenerational trauma and collective trauma aren't interconnected
- Believing that this chapter has nothing to do with you. It does. It's our collective history and we can decide to collectively break cycles.

Reconnecting to Our Roots

One of my clients, Luna, is an Indigenous woman from a mountainous region in Mexico. Her native language was an Indigenous language, and at that time in my career, I was more comfortable with giving therapy in English, but we met in the middle, speaking our common language of Spanish. I was brought on to work with her and her child on family rehabilitation, in order to help keep them from going into the foster care system. She was suspected of hitting her child. Although we could not fully confirm this, we did need to take action to protect her child and help Luna to disengage from this behavior. My aim was to be the liaison who would help her understand why her body was stuck in a historical, collective, and intergenerational nervous system that catapulted her into an explosive rage that her little one would then absorb. I had the added task of helping her understand the cumulative layers related to collective trauma: how our cultures normalize the use of physical punishment of children, how continuing the cycle of collective trauma was not the desire her ancestors had for her, and how her daughter was feeling more disconnected from her culture because the person who most represented her culture, her mother, didn't create a safe and loving atmosphere. Keeping her family close to their roots was really important to Luna. In addition, I understood that a grounded sense of racial and cultural identity was important for her daughter to have, as this acts as a buffer to collective trauma, so I needed to help Luna see that her actions were having the opposite effect. They were disconnecting her child from a rooted sense of identity and a healthy connection with the most important relationship in her life, the one she had with her mother, Luna. So we had work to do.

We had to get to the source of many things in our time together, but we first focused on settling Luna's intergenerational nervous system. In order to change her daughter's behavior without the use of physical punishment, Luna herself had to feel calm enough to be able to communicate her instructions. We all have to focus on settling our own bodies first, before we can transition into adopting different behaviors that have a larger impact.

The second part of our time together was mostly educational, where

Luna and I were able to learn how the collective trauma of Indigenous and Afro-Indigenous people, matched with the further traumas she suffered as an immigrant in the US, was implicated in her anger-driven actions. This was a lot for her to absorb. Since she needed some coping skills she could lean on, we bolstered her generational resilience in the same ways you are learning to do in the Breaking the Cycle practices of this book. She and I did a lot of nervous system restoration. We shared meals in session, she brought us Mexican hot chocolate so we could commune over the drink during one of our sessions, and I offered her a journal with a map of her homeland on it so that she could remember her mission to stay rooted. We were creating a holistic environment for her anger to safely exist, be felt, and be released. We were doing so by honoring the positive parts of the culture and releasing the parts that perpetuated emotional injury.

Luna and I then integrated her child into treatment. She was able to hear from her child how Luna made her feel when she screamed at her or when she grabbed her slipper to instigate fear and demand respect. Her child once said in a family session, with tears in her eyes, "I'm scared of you." I asked Luna to look into her child's teary eyes and tell me if that pain looked familiar. She said, "Yes, she's me." What Luna referenced in that moment was the way she was able to see her own inner child wounds in her daughter. She saw her intergenerational inner child. This was the first moment when she could see a long lineage of collective pain all at once. Her anger and masked cultural norms hadn't previously allowed her to see that familiar pain. And that was enough for her to decide to break the cycle and help others in her family to do the same.

Breaking the Cycle: Disrupting Collective Trauma

In the same ways I recommended that Luna and I start with settling her intergenerational nervous system, I will suggest you seek to do that for yourself as an important step toward disrupting collective trauma. In doing so, you will be releasing the remnants of the collective pain that live in you. Head back to the Breaking the Cycle exercise in chapter 6, and if you can, integrate that practice into your daily routine to help settle your nervous system on an ongoing basis.

When you're ready to take an added step toward community healing, I would recommend you shift into action that focuses on collective rehabilitation at a local level first, and then consider how you may expand your work more globally.

When dealing with something as personal as intergenerational trauma, it can be easy to forget that we are all a part of a greater whole. When we can see trauma on a larger scale, in the ways that we have in this chapter, it helps us humanize each other's experiences and motivates us to contribute to the minimization of external trauma factors for the greater society, for our collective peace. Disrupting the cycles of collective trauma will take all our collective efforts. It will take community action to help those most disenfranchised by these trauma systems. And it will take advocacy to break down the values and practices that keep these forms of trauma enshrined in our culture. For those who feel like this is a tall order and aren't sure where to start, you can start locally or virtually. I find that a road map for how to disrupt can be very helpful. Let's consider adopting these upcoming practices so you can start breaking the cycle at the community, societal, or global level and expand your healing out into the world.

This work can also be done in community, so see if you can commission a co-healing partner in one of the areas of communal rehabilitation listed below. This is a moment when doing this work in community could really matter.

Some examples of community rehabilitation could be:

- Helping people in your immediate circle and community to embody greater awareness about how they themselves perpetuate trauma; perhaps your way of doing this is by hosting book clubs in your local community that feature the work of cycle breakers or volunteering at community centers to discuss alternatives to harmful cultural practices (cultural influences), racial-cultural literacy (systemic influences), or literature on how to minimize our carbon footprint (natural influences)

- Helping develop greater identity consciousness (e.g., racial consciousness, body consciousness, etc.) in the children in your life by having them read culturally affirming books that promote healthy cultural saliency, while supporting them in taking age-appropriate steps toward equity

- Resharing the information of a local organization that works on securing resources for communities you wish to help, or even helping them build their marketing materials or outreach efforts

- Lobbying for bills that help protect children who live in homes where they have a high risk of experiencing intergenerational ACEs; perhaps the bills you focus on are those that can help establish healthier homes for the entire family unit, so that the children and parents can embody intergenerational liberation from their own pain and become cycle breakers themselves

- Initiating community circles with other people who share a similar story and can feel validated by the stories of your shared ancestors

- Supporting or donating to social institutions already doing good community work that you can stand by

- Providing community members with the tools that are known to be effective, so that they can facilitate their own liberation and not have to rely on others to liberate them; you can start by sharing this book, financial literacy texts, texts that shed light on modern-day racial caste systems, books that disrupt heteronormativity, books that emphasize body positivity, books that shed light on ableist ideologies and practices, and any other book or resource that can expand and liberate minds

Remember that you can create your own justice, whatever that may look like; it is valid, enough, and will have an intergenerational impact.

What You've Learned So Far

In this chapter, you explored how intergenerational trauma has collective roots. You learned more about the experiences of collective crisis, how severe social stress impacts the collective, and how to disrupt societal messages and practices that keep trauma patterns filtering into our homes. You were then guided through actionable steps toward breaking cycles at different levels of collective trauma. It can be difficult to digest information that has a lot of layers like what you learned in this chapter. So I encourage you to pause, reflect, breathe, and honor your own collective trauma prior to heading into the next chapter, where you will be focusing on grief.

REFLECTION QUESTIONS

How has it been for you to add this dimension of trauma to the lens of how you see generational pain?

What was the most difficult part of reading this chapter? Where did you feel it in your body?

What made you feel most enlightened after reading this chapter?

Where do you feel most inclined to do collective rehabilitation work?

PART 3

Alchemizing Your Legacy

CHAPTER 10

Grieving Your Traumatic Lineage

Give yourself permission to let go of the past and step out of your history.

—Oprah Winfrey

Now that you've come to understand the full spectrum of factors, both internal and external, that contribute to keeping cycles of intergenerational trauma going, it's time that you start the process of shedding. Shedding the pain will help make way for healing to take root. This won't necessarily call for you to discard your relationships with family members, although that is also very welcome, if needed. This process of shedding is more comprehensive than that. It's a process of shedding antiquated expectations of who your family could have been, old ideas of who you thought you were, and expired perceptions of the world around you. It's a moment to step into a new reality, one where you are able to live authentically and see things for what they truly are: both hurtful and survivable.

Breaking cycles requires digging into the family shadows and acknowledging the mental health issues that different family members have been suffering from. It means shoveling through the dirt to find the ways in which each person has learned to absorb pain and the ways they perpetuate shame and keep these shame cycles tucked inside the closet of family secrets. It requires telling it like it is and disrupting the ways things have been. It requires a reconciliation with the fact that the way family members recall events will be vastly different from what you remember. You may remember them being deeply depressed and neglectful of your emotional needs. They may recall being fully present and attending to your emotional needs for the entirety of your childhood. You may recall that a grandparent hit you repeatedly when you got bad grades, while their recollection was of having calm conversations with you about how you could improve your studying skills.

The stories will clash. As a cycle breaker, you'll find that some family members will try to rewrite history in order to escape responsibility. They may gaslight you into questioning the way events took place. This can lead you into doubting yourself. Family members might shun you for airing the family's dirty laundry and make you feel guilty for stepping out of generations of trauma. As a result, you may very well be triggered and retraumatized as you shed family shame.

Accepting that this is likely to be a painful process will help prepare your heart for the disappointment that could come up. That's right, more grief! You'll have to let go of the fantasy that one day you will be fully heard by those who have hurt you, that certain family members will change their behavior, and that things will be notably different as soon as your cycle-breaking work begins. Delaying rejection of this fantasy can complicate your grief and shame. Accepting that this *is* fantasy can be liberating. It's time to grieve and let go. It's time to step into a new way of being. If you're ready, then let's continue.

Intergenerational Loyalty

We humans gravitate toward what we know because the unknown is terrifying. We don't do well with uncertainty, even if what's on the other side has the potential to be better for us. This explains why grieving is so hard. You are pushed into an unknown. When you lose people in your life, you have to sit with the uncertainty of how life will be without them. Intergenerational healing, however, calls you to wholeheartedly step into the unknown and leave behind what's been familiar. It calls us to shake our Intergenerational Trauma Tree and allow the rotting leaves to fall. It requires acceptance of those fallen leaves and the trauma responses that they held within them. However, humans don't do well with letting the unhealthy family tree leaves fall, with evolution, or with the unknown. Emotionally, we crave what we know. We crave the familiar: familiar people, familiar patterns, familiar behaviors. Even when the familiar is something that hurts us, we gravitate toward it. We repeat it. That's why many of us stay in dysfunction. We stay tied to family bonds that, albeit hurtful, can feel comforting because they are predictable and keep us from facing uncertainty.

To add a layer to this dilemma, many of us feel that leaving a family behind, even a dysfunctional one, means not only abandoning them but abandoning ourselves. The sentiment that keeps us in those family dynamics no matter the consequence is what I call *intergenerational loyalty*. It's the self-sacrifice that we make in order to stay close to our families. It's a way to synchronize with them, keep things as they are. It's an energetic entanglement. This sense of loyalty makes it doubly hard to leave behind family environments defined by toxicity and chaos. You were socialized to stay in the cycle, not to disrupt it, so intergenerational loyalty has been all you've known.

Many cycle breakers are taught to maintain this loyalty by keeping up appearances and presenting a pulled-together family facade. This means you're preprogrammed to carry family secrets, maintain dysfunction, and keep the cycle intact. Keeping family secrets is learned behavior. Sometimes, that behavior is rooted in cultural beliefs around not airing your family's "dirty laundry" and comes from valuing privacy and avoiding shame. The fear is that your dirty laundry might bring humiliation onto your family by casting them in a negative light and inviting in judgment. A common phrase found in South Asian communities in reference to this is "log kya kahenge," which in Urdu and Hindu languages translates to "What will people think?" The unsaid rule here is that you don't bring embarrassment upon your family. Those who wish to go against this value and discuss family business outwardly risk being cast out.

And although some public proclamations of what happened to you can offer temporary relief, shedding intergenerational loyalty isn't about broadcasting all your family's shame to the world. It is instead about courageously having ongoing conversations about these secrets, with yourself, and maybe even with your family members themselves. It's about getting curious and asking questions like "Can we have a conversation about grandma's lifelong battle with depression and how her depressive anger was hurtful?" It's about calling out the elephant in the room and clearing out the unaddressed tensions that have always clouded your home.

Bringing these hidden layers out requires time and work. It requires patience. It requires giving these secrets a voice, rather than keeping them quiet. Silence is rarely an effective strategy for healing lineage trauma, because even if you are able to stifle the suffering by keeping quiet, it will creep up in later generations. And the impact becomes more powerful with each generation of silence. If you keep the diseased part of the family tucked away, it will only continue to fester and mature, until eventually it infects each one of its members. Therefore, the more you unearth those secrets that keep your lineage diseased, the less control that trauma has over your family.

However, it's important to always temper your expectations when unearthing generations of secrets and shame. This work is complex. Healing doesn't happen in one neat conversation, but in repeated messy conversations, persistent confrontations of those secrets, and holding firm to your cycle-breaking practices. In some cases, it won't be possible to have meaningful conversations or achieve reconciliation with family members who have also maintained the cycle. When that happens, you must pivot your efforts and protect yourself first. Even though it feels like you're leaving others behind to continue in pain while you shed those layers, you must face the loss from discarding your loyalty.

Your own reflections about family secrets may lead you to realize that you have also contributed to secret keeping. Many cycle breakers find themselves realizing the same, so it's safe to say that you're not alone in this conundrum. It's very common for cycle breakers to have first been cycle keepers. The realization that you may have contributed to maintaining your family's cycle of trauma can be the step that finally allows you to shift gears, to fully grieve your cycle-keeping identity.

The hard truth is that you can't heal your own intergenerational wounds while wallowing in the shame of your contributions to intergenerational pain. If you didn't know it was a symptom of intergenerational trauma, you didn't know to stop it. Instead, you must shift your own mindset to the present and the future in order to liberate yourself from any hold the past has had on you. So if you're there, wallowing and feeling the shame, hold your heart tight, breathe as needed, and remember that you're not alone in this. Many cycle breakers across the globe face the same issue when breaking the cycle. What you can do now is acknowledge this new understanding of your own intergenerational loyalty and disrupt your allegiance to shame.

Remember that generational agreement you tore up in chapter 1? This is a healthy moment to check back in with the new agreement you created and recommit to breaking the cycle. This layer of your shedding will require your full dedication, because the work of shedding shame and secrets can feel especially challenging. I can assure you, however, that breaking up with the past will be a worthwhile step.

Breaking Up with Shame

Shame is the idea that you are bad, broken, or inadequate. It is a negative self-appraisal that causes a deep, painful feeling of humiliation and distress. Shame is also highly prevalent among trauma sufferers and one of the core emotions that we must address when undoing trauma.

In order to step into your intergenerational higher self, you'll have to cut through the forest of shame that intergenerational trauma has left you with. When you break up with shame, you're cutting ties with the main emotion that has kept you in cycles. You're leaving behind your comfort zone. Breaking up with those feelings means introducing discomfort and the possibility of a full existential crisis. When you invite in this type of worldview-altering work, you take the chance to find yourself again, or maybe even for the first time. Developing that new identity, one with a healthier relationship to your lineage, can feel lonely and heartbreaking.

Shame emerges when a person starts to believe that something is globally wrong with them. That they're flawed, unlovable, and lacking in worth. It's the belief that you are too much, too little, or too insignificant. Shame is a global negative self-evaluation that leaves you feeling both powerless and worthless. Shame is what happens when a child or adult yearns to be seen and cared for but instead is met with rejection, disdain, judgment, and humiliation. When left unaddressed, shame becomes a lifelong burden. It leads to avoidant, self-destructive, and reckless behavior, and disrupts a person's capacity to properly regulate their emotions and emotional responses.

It's also an emotion that can be easily passed on to others. Children especially bear the brunt of their parents' shame because they're an accessible target to displace shame onto. When people in our lives, especially caregivers, don't assume responsibility for their actions, especially if they didn't do so when we were kids, the natural developmental response is to feel personal responsibility and internalize shame. Prior to adolescence, we don't have abstract thinking skills, so we tend to see things in black or white, this or that, good or bad binaries. As a result, children who are raised in toxic households don't have the ability to see the pain in their homes as the symptom of harmful adult behaviors or intergenerational grief. It's a concept that is far too complex for a child to comprehend. Instead, they internalize those issues as their own and develop a self-narrative that implies they are the ones who are causing the issues. That they are the ones who are at fault.

It's normal for a child to believe that their parent can't possibly be bad. This is mostly because of how hard it is for a child to integrate into their underdeveloped mind that a parent can have harmful qualities yet still love them. Again, it's a concept far too abstract for a child to intuitively grasp. And so, a child will assume that if the parent is the *good person*, but *bad things* are happening, then the only possible *bad person* is the child. They think, "My parent is a good person, so I must be the bad kid that's making them angry." This leaves them justifying the pain they experience as their own fault and believing they deserved it. The result for that child is a deeply rooted sense of shame. That displacement becomes intergenerational, passed from parent to child.

If your family didn't acknowledge or apologize for their harmful actions, you became the intergenerational bearer of shame and grief. When you dig deeper into your healing, however, you will come to see that this shame isn't yours. That shame has been an expression of repressed grief and emotions that were handed over to you. That grief, when processed, can lead to a resolution of generations of shame living in you.

Shame is always a heavy topic to dive into, so notice what comes up in your body as you sit with all this. What emotions arise? Does it feel

like grief? Is sadness coming up for you? Is there profound rage that
feels too volatile to approach? Do you feel confusion, loss, or a lack of
clarity? All of these are natural responses to sitting with your shame.
Pause here if you need to sit with your personal experience of shame for
a minute. It's important to allow your mind and body to catch up to
what you're reading and to process things slowly and intentionally. If it
helps, say the following to yourself: "I release the generational shame
I've internalized and I replace it with compassion and grace." When
you're ready, dive back in to keep learning.

Healing Their Pain

You are already healing a significant part of your lineage by healing
yourself. Your decision to break cycles is going to have ripple effects
on your family and community, because when you show up more
healed, others have to adjust their way of being around you, which
means they feel the effects of healing too. You disrupt patterns by simply existing as a more healed self. However, some cycle breakers have an
essential desire to help their families and communities heal too.

Having a desire to heal people in one's family is different from having a *duty* to their healing. If you're feeling a sense of duty, that could
be remnants of savior fantasies from childhood. Children of immature
parents, as well as children of parents who use substances, feel a duty to
rescue their parent. That's because in the past, those children have actually had to rescue them. It is not your responsibility to heal anyone but
yourself, especially if you feel it would be dangerous or even just emotionally too heavy to do so. Give yourself permission to move on alone
if you know in your heart that these conversations will lead only to
more pain. If, however, you feel that you'd like to introduce your family
members to these topics, then read ahead for some tools for navigating
these difficult conversations.

Having Conversations About Intergenerational Trauma

Every time Brooklyn hit a milestone in treatment, she wanted to help her family apply her learning to their own trauma responses. In part, this response was based on a sense of duty Brooklyn felt to help them. But she was also motivated by her desire to build a home that reflected the same peace *externally* that she was working to obtain *internally* in therapy. "I feel so defeated when I go home," she would say in sessions when her attempts to keep her peace at home failed. She felt defeated when she would try to guide her family to change by helping them adopt the same methods that were helping her change. Her efforts were unsuccessful. Upon reflecting on her frustrations in session, we noticed a pattern in the way she approached her family members on this topic.

When initiating conversations about generational trauma, Brooklyn often started by telling her family all the ways they had hurt her. It's instinctive for people to get defensive when they are blamed. That's an example of a survival response. Brooklyn's approach would halt productive conversation and any possibility for healing right from the beginning. When she pointed the finger at one of her family members, it brought up deep shame for them both. Brooklyn needed her family to be open and vulnerable, but instead their defenses went up. Once we had identified the issue, Brooklyn and I set a primary goal. We needed to work on the delivery so that she could have greater success with her message being heard, especially by her mother.

To get started, we needed to identify Brooklyn's mom's level of willingness to participate in a healing conversation with her daughter. Brooklyn *most* wanted to have these conversations with her mom, but because she had been so traumatized by her mom, she didn't know where to start. We decided Brooklyn should wait for a moment when their intergenerational window of tolerance was open and inviting, because they would both be calmer and more settled. First, they would do an activity that could help increase their bond. One of their shared rituals was eating ice cream and watching a game show on TV. They loved doing that together, so it was a healthy starting point. When they were both more settled, Brooklyn's second task was to offer an entry into the conversation. We walked through some reminders for Brooklyn, so that she could approach her mom (and herself) with gentleness. The reminders were:

- Remember that these conversations are breaking decades, and sometimes centuries, of unhelpful communication patterns and dynamics.
- Remember that the intergenerational nervous system will be activated in both of your bodies as you dialogue.
- Remember that people will only be able to have these conversations at their level of healing.
- Remember that these conversations can happen only as long as they continue to be emotionally digestible to both parties.
- As soon as the conversation pushes beyond anyone's intergenerational window of tolerance, you may see more trauma responses manifest in the conversation, and you may start seeing those psychological defenses building up, leaving you feeling unheard and invalidated, which is the opposite result of what you desire.
- Be willing to abandon the conversation or even the desire to have the conversation, if the other party does not show mutual willingness to heal and connect

Next, we used a skill I call DRIVE, which would place Brooklyn in the driver's seat of the conversations so that she could maneuver more smoothly in order to achieve the outcome of being heard. DRIVE is an acronym that stands for Don't point fingers, Relay a short and digestible message, Initiate with emotion, Visualize your intergenerational nervous system, and Exercise action.

- **Don't Point Fingers**—Finger pointing will backfire about 100 percent of the time. When a person feels blamed, their psychological defenses get kicked up, and they will defend themselves. This will surely leave you feeling invalidated and retriggered. Be mindful of your need to place blame, and resist it. Instead, focus on what I call the *issues and tissues* (the actual problem you would like to fix and the emotions that it brings up for you).

- **Relay a Short and Digestible Message**—When we're having a difficult conversation with someone, we tend to speak at length because we become so eager to tell the other person everything at once. Once we feel brave enough to start a hard conversation, we want to capitalize on that bravery while we can. But slow and steady wins the race. Place one issue on the table in as few words as possible. Pause and let the person digest what you're saying before calling out the emotions that this one issue evokes in you. This works best, because when we're having difficult conversations, our nervous system response can suppress our cognitive brain's functions. So, the shorter the message, the greater the chance of it being heard and digested.

- **Initiate with Emotion**—When you state the emotions that you feel, the conversation will be more feelings-based and you will find it easier to shift away from blaming. Focusing on emotions allows you both to humanize each other and see each other more deeply.

- **Visualize Your Intergenerational Nervous System**—Remember that through this conversation, two nervous systems are internalizing and reacting. Both of those nervous systems are intergenerationally linked and come with long, layered histories. Consider this when you see emotions starting to flare up. Take a gentle look into yourself and notice any cues that you may be in a fight, flight, freeze, or fawn response, and if so, consider your next move, regulating, pausing, or continuing. Regulating or pausing will help you settle better and prepare you to more effectively continue.

- **Exercise Action**—This conversation is about moving forward, so propose one solution that the two of you could employ *today* to help you start moving forward from the issue. Remember to keep it short and accessible so that you can both actually do it.

Some people feel more at ease when they have a starting point, so sometimes I'll role-play how to set up the conversation with clients. The setup we initiate tends to sound something like this:

- "I'm hoping to have a discussion about something that's really important to me. Are you willing to sit with me for a few moments?"
- If yes, "Before we begin, I understand that my automatic response with difficult conversations is to lash out; I've noticed that yours is to shut down. Do you think we can both commit to be present and compassionate with each other here?" (This places the responsibility on you both and shifts away from pointing fingers.)
- If yes, "I've felt I haven't received the level of love I've needed." (This is how a message can be relayed in a short and direct way, using "I" statements and not pointing fingers.)
- Then pause and say, "It makes me a bit anxious to share this, but how are you feeling about what I just said?" (This can be how to integrate emotion-centered language in relation to your experience and theirs.)

- If things start to sour, you can say, "I am noticing that we both are a little uneasy. Can we pause and continue the conversation after we've caught a breath?" (This would be how to attend to the intergenerational nervous system, because you are noticing the cues of fight, flight, freeze, or fawn, and choosing to settle your intergenerational nervous systems with a breath, rather than continue to push it into overdrive.)

- If you see you're both ready to continue, you can shift into action with a statement like, "I would like to propose that we start saying the words *I love you* to one another." (This is a short, tangible solution you can both start today.)

- "Can we try it now? I'll start: I love you." (This can be how to initiate the solution in order to break the ice.)

- Lead with feelings and gratitude for their willingness to participate in the conversation with you. "Thank you for sitting with me to discuss this. I know this hasn't been easy. This conversation has meant a lot to me."

- Notice any urges to tie the conversation neatly with a bow, and sit with the discomfort of the conversation being different from your fantasy of what would happen or what you anticipated the end result would be.

- Remember to take deep breaths as you exit the conversation and invite them to do the same, so that your intergenerational nervous systems can reestablish a sense of safety and peace.

- Repeat these conversations as many times as is needed, with healthy breaks in between for both of you to process what you cover.

- Most of all, temper your expectations. You may not receive an "I love you" back or whatever solution you proposed. You may not even get to relay your message. The conversation could be cut short and the entire plan could dissipate. That's OK. Still, focus on how you feel about the lack of resolution, because your feelings are valid here. And give space for you to also feel pride in yourself for approaching a difficult dialogue with so much intention.

- And if you choose to not have any conversation that looks like this, know that this is also OK. You don't have to force yourself into conversations that may not resolve the patterns you wish to break. You can instead choose to shift away from the unhealthy dynamics and work on yourself and your health.

Healing conversations are undoubtedly some of the most difficult we will have in this lifetime. Each conversation has the power to create microsolutions toward the larger goal of building legacies of wellness instead of pain. In having these conversations, you may not be able to completely dissolve the pain your loved ones have carried or the pain they have caused you. This is an especially important reminder for those who have suffered deep, complex trauma and for whom reconciliation is not ideal or possible. Whether you are choosing to have the conversation or you have determined that it's not worth trying, writing down your emotions about your decision is always good practice. Here, grab your journal and try writing about the people you'd like to have these conversations with. Maybe go so far as to imagine what the beginnings of this conversation might look like with one of them. Making a plan can be powerful step toward initiating a conversation that you've been holding back on for years.

Leaving Behind Intergenerational Guilt

Let me help illustrate how a DRIVE conversation can go with an example from my own family. My mother worked tirelessly to provide for us while also sending money back to the DR each month to her mother and her seven siblings. Her dollar had to stretch so far. And despite her thirty-plus years of trying, she could never get us above the poverty line.

She did a lot with the little she made as a hairdresser, but we would always hear her talk about how much more she wished she could have done.

Over the years, my sister, father, and I have had conversations with my mother that follow the DRIVE model, in order to help her internalize a different narrative, one in which she sees how much she has done for our entire family. Our end goal here was to help her transition from her stuck place, her guilt, into a place of pride and peace. We also wanted guilt to be released from our family, since we often carried this guilt with her. After years of these conversations, only recently have I heard her reflect on how proud she has been that she could help her family, especially during her mother's last days on earth. And although some might not see so small a comment as a revolutionary step forward, to us, hearing her speak those words was monumental. This was the small impact we had the power to make. I couldn't change my mother's past, all the guilt and what suffering poverty, migration, family disruptions, sexism, classism, and racism had cost her. We couldn't change our family's past burdens and hurt, but we *could* teach each other to think differently about those circumstances beyond our control. We could celebrate the small victories and grieve the rest. We could release the burdening parts of our Intergenerational Trauma Tree and keep what felt healthy. This was how we would shake our own family tree and allow the leaves that reflected intergenerational guilt to fall. I see peace in my mother and that brings me peace. It has not been a perfectly peaceful life beyond this and I have had to resolve my own grief about having to hold so much emotional space for my parents who couldn't find their own resolutions in time for it to reach the rest of us. But the peace that my mother in particular has been able to obtain later in life has been enough for me. That peace has become intergenerational, meaning we have both experienced some level of comfort. This serenity has replaced some of the layered guilt we have carried for decades. This is what I hope you'll be able to also do: use DRIVE where needed and process the grief of what you could not change.

You Don't Have to Forgive the Hurt

Forgiveness is not a requisite to breaking cycles of trauma. It never has been and it never will be. Many times, I'm asked by clients or during talks if it is necessary to exculpate the people who have hurt us in order to heal ourselves. The short answer is no. This is in no way necessary. Some people won't be deserving of your forgiveness and that's OK. Other times, you won't have the desire, motivation, or even capacity to offer forgiveness and that is also OK. Some things are simply unforgivable. Some people have been so deliberate in causing harm or choosing to stay in harmful cycles that leaning on forgiveness will just leave room for them to continue bringing pain into your life. In these cases, forgiveness won't bring about any type of resolution that can help your healing path. It can instead add more emotional weight to an already heavy experience that you have to sort through. So, if pardoning that person is something that you don't see happening, honor that for yourself, instead of pushing yourself in the direction of exonerating someone from their behaviors just because you believe that you must. You don't have to make allowances for anyone in your life. And you can even love them and still not condone what they did or continue to do. For example, you can have a parent whose emotionally immature behavior manifests as guilt-tripping. They manipulate you into doing things for them at your own expense and spiral you into feeling shame for giving into their tactics. You resent that they continue to trigger you and loop you back into the same cycles that you are trying so hard to break. You can decide to create a healthy distance between yourself and your parent and not forgive their manipulative behaviors. You can break the cycle and also not forgive. Both can happen simultaneously. That is to say, you are still a cycle breaker if you choose to not let someone off the hook. Some cycle breakers choose this path, because it offers them greater peace. And so can you. It is a valuable approach to healing and many times it is the only way forward. Instead of spending energy trying to force yourself into excusing others, you can lay to rest the idea of forgiving and instead allow yourself to grieve the reconciliation you wish you could have had.

Attending Their Funeral

For my clients and in my personal life, I always push for change and disruption that can produce healing. I especially push for this, because cutting ties with people may sometimes be essential, but when overdone, it can perpetuate profound loneliness that can be even more detrimental to your health. Having difficult dialogues, like Brooklyn had with her mother or like we had with my mother, is a part of how we can produce healing that forges healthier connections with our loved ones, instead of pushing ourselves too far into a toxic loneliness. These conversations can create microshifts that have a profound impact and are typically worthwhile. So if the opportunity is there, yes, move in the direction of change and resolution, but if the opportunity is not possible, because it's far too consequential and dangerous, or if a resolution is simply not possible, you have to take a different approach. This approach is more internal. This approach requires grief. The truth is that for many of the relationships you have, you won't be able to change the status quo. And for many traumatized people, this is a tough pill to swallow. Cycle breakers share a common desire to go back and change things and can come to see that change isn't happening, which is deeply disheartening. In the moments when change in others isn't an option, change in yourself should be the goal. If you find that this is far too hard for you to do, there's a likely chance that you're stuck in the grief stage of denial. You are delaying the inevitable loss that awaits when you have to either let go of someone or let go of the ideas you held about them. Cycle breakers often have to walk away from family members without an apology, without their love, and without their acknowledgment of how they passed down pain. You'll have to sit with the anger, sadness, denial, chaos, and depression that it causes to fully accept that. A person who inflicted pain may pass away without ever apologizing for their toxic behavior. And as a cycle breaker, you have to candidly ask yourself, "How will I deal with that reality?" It will be important to decide if you will be willing to let go of those old expectations to one day hear their remorse or spend years waiting for something that may never happen. Coming to terms with grief means dealing with the deeply saddening cards that you've been dealt. Ancestral healing requires you to release those traumatic retentions, shadows, and unmanifested desires that left behind hurt. And it means that you commit to no longer involuntarily fighting the internal battles of others.

In order to do this, you will have to lay to rest the family you thought you had, meaning that you'll need to leave behind all expectations of the family you wished for but never had; I call this your *false family*. It's the family you thought you knew before having the full picture and truly seeing your family with all their flaws and shortcomings. It's the idea of family you held on to before you were awakened to these generational truths. Now that you've been more enlightened about these truths, you have an opportunity to welcome in your new reality and welcome in what I call your *true family*: the family that you actually have, the one that is flawed, sometimes hurtful, maybe toxic, filled with their own pain, and intergenerationally wounded. It's the family that you see in front of you now that the veil has been lifted.

Once you're able to see all the layers of trauma that each person carries, you see them truthfully, honestly, and without a filter. You see their true selves. That's your true family, meaning this is the real family you've been given. The family that can be hurtful and has indeed caused you to experience emotional turmoil. And coming to terms with who your true family is requires letting go of the old ways you saw them. It's a journey of loss. It's like attending an internal funeral of the people you lost, people who only existed in your mind, because they were never real. They were false representations of the true family in front of you. If you're hoping to learn how to take yourself through the loss of your false family, let's get into the practice of letting go.

Breaking the Cycle: Letting Go of the Family You Wish You Had

Moving out of a harmful status quo and into an intergenerational legacy will require a transition through grief. Sometimes the hardest thing to shed is the wish of what could have been. The wish that you could have been born without trauma. That you could have been loved differently by family. That you could have belonged to a family that dealt with their hurt before this generation. That you could have been born into a society that didn't reinforce emotional hurt. You could been, but weren't. And that is profoundly hard to digest. As a way to transition from this place of stuckness and grief, I'd like to offer a practice I call Saying Goodbye. We are going to be drafting a goodbye letter to your false family.

To help you settle into your practice, head to your safe place to write. Have your writing materials handy but also any items that can bring you comfort and ground you. Gather your breath, and if it feels right to you, take three deep inhales with closed eyes. Once you've taken the third breath, know that it's time to start letting go.

You're ready for this, so let's begin.

- First consider whether this letter will be dedicated to one person or multiple people.
- Address your letter with their name(s).
- And begin with this: "I am on a quest toward honoring myself. I am shifting what I am devoting this life to. And that is toward

building an intergenerational legacy. But I can't do this until I let go of the heavy burdens I've been holding on to. So I write this letter to let go of the intergenerational burdens that have plagued me, and you."

Now transition into identifying what you're letting go of in this way:

- Name what you wish they did (e.g., I wish you had told me you loved me).
- Name what they *actually* did (e.g., but instead you withheld the verbal expressions of love, which I needed).
- Name the intergenerational thread to their behavior (e.g., perhaps because you never had a solid model for verbalizing love).
- Name what you're willing to take with you (e.g., I will take with me the moments when I saw you trying to show me love through actions, even if you could never say the words).
- Name what you're going to let go of (e.g., I will let go of this deep-rooted desire to hear you say the words, "I love you, my child").
- Name what you will replace this void with (e.g., I will instead say the words to myself every single day).
- Name how this will be legacy building (e.g., my love will have a ripple effect on my life and the next generation).
- Now take the letter and place it somewhere where you can reread it when you need a reminder of the love you deserve, and the work you have done.
- Take the moment you need to sit with this practice.
- Transition from it with deep breaths and by giving yourself a tight hug.
- Pour hugs into yourself for the rest of the day and take it easy—this was hard!
- And congratulations on completing this critical task.

What You've Learned So Far

In this chapter, you explored the concept of intergenerational loyalty. You were able to gather an understanding of how courageous conversations, rather than continued secret keeping and shame, are the real acts of devotion to family and to yourself. Part of this journey requires a necessary step of grieving, so you were taught the importance of transitioning from the family that you once believed you had (your false family) to the family you now know you have (your true family). You learned how this type of loss is processed in the mind, body, and spirit, and how it needs to be honored in the same ways we honor those who are no longer with us. Just as with any loss and grief you've had to process in your life, this grief work can leave you feeling heavy, so be sure to offer yourself a gentle break; perhaps make some lemongrass tea or do some intergenerational EFT tapping to rebalance. Release is important for this work, so give yourself a moment to let go before diving into the next section on generational resilience.

REFLECTION QUESTIONS

How was it for you to reflect on your false family versus your true family?

How was it for you to release the need to heal their pain?

What came up for you as you completed the Breaking the Cycle practice of saying goodbye?

What's your vision for how life could be once you've let go of these burdens?

CHAPTER 11

Embodying Generational Resilience

I . . . got royalty inside my DNA.

—Kendrick Lamar

Increasing your generational resilience will require that you push yourself in the direction of growth. Intergenerational resilience refers to the endurant strength, healing, and adaptation of the people that we descend from and the ways in which, in our lifetime, we have inherited and built upon their strength to prevail within our own circumstances. As we covered in chapter 2, on your intergenerational higher self, this type of resilience offers you an ability to use individual and collective strengths to live a life that is fuller and more present. It reflects your capacity to bounce back because you embody intergenerational fortitude. When you learn about the strength of your ancestors, you are emboldened. You are able to capture the strength that's been passed down and find the resilience that already lies within you.

Intergenerational resilience is based on not just your own wisdom and strength but also that of your ancestors. It's the wisdom they have left you with, based on how they learned to navigate hardship. It's a type of resilience that crosses time and dimensions and includes all their combined efforts toward survival, from generation to generation. This genetic inheritance is reflected not only in your ingrained trauma responses or emotional vulnerabilities that we've learned about through these chapters; this is a resilience that is reflected in how you have been able to, despite the numerous recycled trauma responses reflected in your Intergenerational Trauma Tree, use innate strength to help you manage through stressful circumstances so that your life doesn't feel like an everlasting obstacle course. It's even reflected in the fact that you've picked up this book and worked on increasing your intergenerational window of tolerance, decreasing your shame, balancing your body, and all the different resilience-building exercises that you've been adopting so far. And it's in all the additional things that you already do in your daily life that have made you an intergenerational trauma survivor and a cycle breaker.

Intergenerational resilience can also be understood from a biological perspective. Epigenetic changes related to trauma aren't all tragic. In fact, they are said to also biologically prepare us to survive the types of traumas that our parents and ancestors had to go through. This is transmissible information that helps us prepare for life by making us both biologically and socially equipped for those similar stressors. You use that innate readiness daily, but you're probably not pausing enough to notice it. Let's take this moment to do just that, to notice how this inheritance of resilience shows up in your daily life.

Think of a recent minor hardship that you've had to overcome. Picture it in your mind. Now picture what you did to get through that circumstance. Take a pause here. What came to mind? Perhaps you pictured how you used your strong problem-solving skills, or how you shifted your perspective on the issue to see it from a different angle, or perhaps you started approaching the hurdle as a learning opportunity. Whatever your version of resilience was for that situation, it stemmed from you and your innate capacities. You were prepared to survive it.

A beautiful thing about generational resilience is also that you can continue building on top of it. You can help promote even more resilience in your mind and body to increase the fortitude that is already there. You can look at your Intergenerational Trauma Tree and at the fortitude that people have had in your lineage and communities, despite the trauma responses held in that tree. This can be another moment to pause and think about how, despite the layered pain, your lineage tree continued to grow. And more specifically, this can be a moment to reflect on the generational gifts offered in your lineage, even though pain was present.

Just as your ancestors and family members did, perhaps more unconsciously than you are doing now, you have the capacity to rehabilitate your body and brain. While they very likely had to rely solely on intuition to repair the stress in their lives, you can build your strength through holistic strategies to reverse the damage of early stress. Ongoing healing practices, like the ones you're learning here, can change your brain and create new neural connections that fire in your favor, rather than against you. Meditation, for example, has been shown to activate brain areas involved in self-regulation, problem solving, healthy behaviors, and interoception (your capacity to be better attuned to your internal states). The more you engage in these practices, the more you will be able to embody resilience. As you continue to read, hold on to the understanding that you have not only an abundant reservoir of intergenerational resilience but also the capacity to continue to elevate your generational fortitude.

Intergenerational Growth and Abundance

Post-traumatic growth is a process of psychological change and endurance that a person adopts after they've experienced trauma. The concept of post-traumatic growth helps us understand the development of hope and confidence that can, with work, follow a life of traumatic stressors. It is a process in which the person is able to both acknowledge what has happened, like the multiple ways you acknowledged trauma transmissions in your Intergenerational Trauma Healing Assessment, and also develop new meaning in life that focuses on the future. Intergenerational post-traumatic growth works through a similar, yet more layered, lens. It is how we can invite abundance into our lives by way of both our own strength *and* our ancestors' wisdom. Intergenerational post-traumatic growth helps us move beyond our individual selves and see (1) how others have contributed to our wisdom and (2) how we can continue pouring that wisdom into future generations.

There are seven areas that characterize this type of growth. Each features one part of the journey from intergenerational trauma to intergenerational abundance. Taken together, they represent the furthering of intergenerational resilience. And yes, intergenerational resilience can be strengthened on a continuous basis, even when chronic stressors are the norm in your life, like when you hold identities that are marginalized. The more you can embody resilience, the less life's woes can shake you up. Let's look at each of these areas of intergenerational post-traumatic growth, so that you can gather a better sense of what they are. As you read, consider how you may already be adopting some of these practices into your life or how you would like to focus on growing in any particular area.

GENERATING NEW STRENGTH

This area of intergenerational post-traumatic growth refers to your capacity to deal with life's stressors through practices that help your intergenerational nervous system feel more at ease. We've already learned that our nervous systems are created to bounce back from traumas. They are inherently resilient. But since intergenerational trauma causes your nervous system to be in constant overdrive, it experiences wear and tear, the allostatic overload that we learned about in chapter 3. However, you are able to increase your capacity for greater generational resilience by helping your intergenerational nervous system experience more rest and recovery. This means that when you create an opportunity to focus on relaxing, you are training yourself to be even more resilient. You are helping expand your intergenerational window of tolerance. This will serve you individually, by helping you feel more peace in your life, but it also contributes to how you modify your body's biology for the next generation. An added bonus is that the more you settle your nervous system, the more you'll be able to feel connected to others, including the children in your life, which helps them experience adults like yourself in a safe and loving way. You can also help expand your intergenerational window of tolerance with the following practices:

- **Teatime**—Remember the tea breaks and tea sessions I mentioned in chapter 3? Teas, herbs, and botanicals, like chamomile, lavender, lemon balm, and valerian, have been used for ages as traditional stress balms, due to their calming properties. Take time for a mindful tea break, and focus on each step of the tea-making process and savoring the tea slowly. This is a way in which you can introduce a gentle calming moment into your daily life and take inventory of the shifts it produces, while also enjoying the soothing effects of the tea blends you choose.
- **Different Meditations**—The effects of both sitting and active meditation have been notable in helping the nervous system recover. Even a five-minute meditation can be enough to boost your daily mental fortitude. See if you can vary how you meditate each day and find the types of meditations that work best to help heal your soul.
- **Spend Time in Natural Elements**—Spending time in nature can help connect you to its tranquility. Our nervous system is

naturally attuned to our environment, so going back into the elements is a way to help rebalance it and ease your mind. You will quickly see how many earthly miracles exist in each moment, which can foster a sense of peace and help you focus on the present, an often hard task for those bodies living in trauma.

- **Shake It Out**—Tension pockets in your nervous system can be shaken out just by shaking parts of your body. You can do this in whatever way feels right for you, such as through dancing, jumping, running, or simply shaking, but the general goal is to help you release any pent-up energy that your body has captured.

There are so many ways to induce relaxation and restoration in your nervous system. Feel free to get into the practices highlighted here, by integrating these into your daily life in some way, or to add a few of your own that feel more personalized. In appendix C, you can find additional practices that can help. I find that it helps people to start their day with generating strength and resilience. Five minutes a day is sufficient devotion to this daily task, but you can increase it to however much you desire and need.

BUILDING SAFER SOCIAL CONNECTIONS

The second aim is to build safer social connections that are defined by vulnerability and trust. As we've learned, one of the most profound ways in which intergenerational trauma rewires the brain is through our ability to connect to others. Learning to foster healthy social connections is therefore a bridge toward healing. The difference between healthy emotional ties and unhealthy ones can be seen in the presence of vulnerability and trust. But this can be challenging for cycle breakers. However, seeking out people who make you feel psychologically safe can enhance how safe we feel in our own bodies, which in turn contributes to our capacity for trust. You learned in chapter 7 about how a secure attachment can offer a buffer against trauma and help heal your intergenerational inner child. That secure attachment requires trust in others. Relearning to trust starts with small moments of microscopic vulnerabilities that help you widen your intergenerational window of tolerance. This means employing those same strategies I coached Yara through. When doing so, you'll have to push yourself outside your comfort zone, but not so much to completely overwhelm your nervous system. The goal is to push yourself just enough to help you create tiny changes that lead to a greater change over time. Some examples of how you can do this are:

- Telling someone something personal you've never mentioned before (not your biggest and most traumatic experience but something light or moderately stressful)
- Allowing someone to do something for you that you would otherwise do for yourself, to help you train your nervous system to rely on others with small tasks
- Telling someone a small need that you have and leaving room for them to fill that need (like a need for a hug, for example)
- Showing someone an aspect of your personality that you tend to keep hidden (especially if you find yourself showing only parts of you that you think people find digestible)

BUILDING A DIFFERENT TYPE OF APPRECIATION FOR LIFE

The third area refers to how you can build a different type of appreciation for life, with the understanding that life is about much more than a traumatic lineage. For those of us who have felt that trauma has been around every corner of life, it can feel like we *are* our trauma, and nothing more. An overidentification with a trauma narrative can actually become all-consuming, breeding depression and hopelessness. Cultivating a more nuanced view of your life, one that allows you to see all that your life is, can be a healthier way to navigate your post-traumatic narrative. This allows you to create a comprehensive, nuanced, and integrated view of your life that allows both traumatic and peaceful experiences to coexist in one person: you. To that end, it can be helpful for you to consider the narrative that you've been holding on to lately and to question whether you've had a heavy focus on trauma. If that's the case, it will be beneficial to reconstruct your own narrative.

In narrative therapy, a type of therapy that helps people identify alternate stories about their lives to widen their view post-trauma, personal stories are rewritten in order to help empower the storyteller. I'd like to offer an opportunity for you to write a short personal story here. Can you write one page that reflects a balanced narrative of your healing? Start by writing about two things: how intergenerational trauma has been a part of your life and the steps you have taken to become a cycle breaker. This allows you an opportunity to reflect on all the heavy lifting you've already done and take stock of the progress you've made. If you wish to continue writing beyond the one page, consider adding some deeper reflections related to the following questions: What is your healed self able to do that your wounded self couldn't? What new perspectives are you gaining through your healing? What new interests are you discovering? What new ways of living are now possible to you? The task is about seeing things from a balanced perspective and appreciating the pros and cons of your story.

DEVELOPING NEW POSSIBILITIES

The fourth area encourages you to engage in new goals that honor your healed self. A large part of this goal of intergenerational healing is to move you closer to your intergenerational higher self. Remember, the intergenerational higher self is the version of yourself that is more settled, enlightened, and wise, and that engages in a different set of daily practices and routines that honor intergenerational growth and abundance. But you don't just arrive at that wiser self instantly; you build up to that version of you over time. It takes a daily commitment to change, finding and developing new interests, new hobbies, new self-care practices, new anything. Taking these new opportunities expands your horizons in many positive ways. You learn new things, and so you create new neural connections around your learning. You create more capacity to see how much there is to life and find hope in even the smallest things.

I could go on, because the list of possibilities is endless. The important factor to consider here is that you can't look into the future without considering what new adventures the future could hold for you. There are plenty of options, so take this moment as an opportunity to consider what those might be for you. I'll give you a few examples from the therapy room and from my own healing to get you started:

- Learning to cook delicious meals that feed your gut microbiome and the millions of neurotransmitters that live there
- Getting into pottery and ceramics, especially the making of teapots and teacups for your mindful teatime breaks
- Going on hikes and seeing the vastness of nature
- Learning to sew and making new clothing items that fit your personality
- Candlemaking and creating new innovative scents that invite nervous system regulation
- Learning a new language, which improves your cognitive flexibility, a key factor in problem-solving that is often compromised with chronic stress
- Setting a new reading goal of twelve books in twelve months to expand your knowledge of the world
- Learning different ways to meditate (e.g., sitting meditations, yoga, meditations with breathwork, writing meditations, etc.)

The more new habits you focus on, the less energy you will have for the old unhealthy ones that took up too much space in your life.

Think about drafting your own list of possibilities and see where you land.

BECOMING SPIRITUALLY GROUNDED

The fifth area is becoming spiritually grounded, meaning that you are working on bridging healthy connections between yourself and the universal elements of life, including higher powers. Abundant evidence exists of humanity's innate need for connection. Whether you're seeking a connection to God, a divine being, the natural world, the cosmos, ancestors, or the universe, you are seeking a relationship with a power outside yourself. Seeking meaning outside yourself is a fundamental part of the human experience and, therefore, a key to true, holistic healing.

Our connection to universal powers and nature through prayer, meditation, ritual, and faith is not only about belief but wellness. Inviting in spiritual groundedness helps us gather deeper awareness, fully develop meaningful beliefs, and find peace in knowing that forces outside us are working on our behalf. Why do you think it feels so good to believe that God has your back, that moon cycles work in your favor, or that the universe is always seeking balance? We are a part of a larger whole. The more you can connect to that truth, the more grounded you could feel along this journey.

If this is a part of your healing that you are hoping to focus on, consider what aspect of spirituality feels true to you and deepen your relationship with that source. It could mean writing letters to your ancestors or attending congregation services more often, or it could mean knowing your cosmic charts to be better attuned to how natural elements impact you. This is a very personal process, so make it your own. Spend time wherever you wish to grow your spiritual connection. And remember that if you don't wish to focus on this area, it is honored as well.

HELPING OTHERS IN YOUR LINEAGE AND COMMUNITY TO HEAL

The sixth area refers to how you extend help toward your lineage and community. In order to help your lineage and community, try showing up as a more healed self (remember that your healing alone creates shifts in your lineage) or by inviting others to co-heal (which, as I mentioned in the introduction, is optional). However, helping others in your family and in your extended community can be a part of how meaning is made out of the ruins of trauma. This communal view is an aspect of healing work that can add an important dimension to your individual healing. For some cycle breakers, this is the only way they can heal—by extending healing to their larger circle. For others, this feels less central to the work. Both approaches are honored. However, generational trauma is not a single-person experience, so you may want to consider who else can benefit from the type of healing you're undergoing. This can be a friend, a community member, or even a stranger. Some examples of how you can do this include:

- Simply showing up as a more healed version of yourself
- Showing someone the Breaking the Cycle practices you're learning
- Inviting someone to do a deep breathing exercise with you
- Inviting someone to a tea break with you
- Sharing with someone who is struggling how to start difficult conversations using the DRIVE method (see the previous chapter)

Remember that this is to be tailored to you and your own healing needs. As always, make it your own.

HELPING HEAL FUTURE GENERATIONS

The seventh and final area of intergenerational post-traumatic growth is that of helping heal future generations. You are an ancestor in the making, and so the impact you have on the world matters. What you do now can have a multigenerational effect. For many cycle breakers, the idea of positively impacting future generations through the legacy of generational wisdom and resilience is the actual driving force behind their cycle-breaking journey. They see their descendants, like their own children, younger family members, children in their communities, children across the globe, or anyone who is of a future generation, as important to consider in their own healing. It can be a driving force for you too. If that is the case, then it'll be beneficial, much as we've done in several previous exercises, to list how you would like to do this. Start by writing down your answer to this question: "How do I wish to impact my future generations?" and see what you come up with. If you're running short on ideas, here are a few to get you started. You can impact future generations by:

- Teaching them about nervous system regulation as a natural way to take care of themselves, so that they don't have to experience as much suffering as you have
- Creating a relationship with them that is rooted in safety and connection, so that they see you as a safe haven
- Engaging in advocacy that can help create safer environments for them, like safer schools with less bullying or violence, for example
- Modeling behaviors that you know will help them build a healthy self-esteem and a healthy self-concept, like apologizing to them or creating an opportunity for them to talk about emotions
- Investing time in disrupting the systems that dull their light and leave room for trauma to take root
- And so much more

We will cover your intergenerational impact in the upcoming chapter, but for now, continue thinking of ways to tailor your impact to your descendants.

Taken together, these areas help you build generational resilience, wisdom, and abundance. They help you understand that your story doesn't start or end with intergenerational trauma, but that it holds so much more meaning than that. Intergenerational post-traumatic growth is about creating the life you deserve and not allowing intergenerational trauma to be the only notable part of your history.

Embracing the Imperfections

Communities across the world create common languages around resilience that everyone in that community understands at a deep level. Community-based symbolism has reflected strength in communities through history and around the world. For example, in postgenocidal Rwanda, survivors of the genocide and their descendants have adopted culturally specific, resilience-related concepts to help rebuild their community: kwihangana (drawing strength from within), kwongera kubaho (manifesting systems that are affirming), and gukomeza ubuzima (moving in the direction of acceptance and growth). Communities across Rwanda have a shared understanding of both the trauma suffered and the resilience captured in their shared survivorship, which is reflected in this new cultural language they have created.

Members of the Cherokee Nation also have common sayings that are culturally understood to reflect resilience. Wilma Mankiller, the first female chief of the Cherokee Nation, elaborated upon the wisdom of nature in teaching her people about resilience, in noting that a cow runs away from a storm but a buffalo charges toward it, getting through the storm much quicker. Mankiller was asserting that if people stand in the courage of their strength while approaching life's storms, they will see themselves through the issue a lot faster. They might even be reminded of their own strength while facing the challenge.

Another resilience-centered perspective is captured in the Japanese practice called kintsugi, in which people repair broken cracks in pottery with gold. The practice teaches that it's possible to pick up the broken pieces, put them back together, embrace the imperfections, and radiate golden light through it. It is believed that the golden cracks add value to the piece and that, similarly, the metaphorical cracks in our lives also make us more precious. When I first learned of kintsugi, I felt deep sorrow, recalling the precious broken pieces of my grandmother's mug. I had thrown them away, so I didn't believe I could engage in the practice to reconstruct it. But then I remembered that I could rebuild from other things that connect me to her and her wisdom.

A few months after my grandmother's mug shattered and left me heartbroken, my parents brought me back rocks from a river in the DR. The rocks my parents collected there, Larimar, are found in only one place in the world: my grandmother's hometown of Barahona. I decided that I would take my Larimar rocks, polish them, and create a beautiful ceramic art piece in honor of my grandmother's resilience and love. I would create my own kintsugi and include these stones. The practice of creating a ceramic piece from that Larimar allowed me to release the sorrow of losing my grandmother's mug and my perceived lost connection to her, so that I could awaken the power of generational resilience and wisdom in me.

Perhaps you have your own story of alchemy: a story of transformation, of turning pain into gold. Or a story of how you stepped into your own generational power. Perhaps it's that you moved to a new city or country and decided to reconstruct your life. Or maybe your story is one where you shifted careers and stepped into your own courage to make that shift. Or maybe your story is one where you were able to step out of the stigma of mental health and work through your trauma. Whatever your story is, it's worthy of your reflection as you continue the course of your healing.

Breaking the Cycle: Increasing Your Generational Resilience

In the spirit of increasing your generational resilience and moving toward growth, let's work on building better social connections, one of the areas needed for intergenerational post-traumatic growth. You can use this tool to safely expand your own social limits—that means doing something in relationships that could make you feel a tiny bit uncomfortable and pairing it with a relaxation exercise, so you can learn to tolerate the discomfort. The relaxation exercise also helps you expand your intergenerational window of tolerance in order to help you foster those deeper connections. I'll offer you a gentle exercise to try that I call Surviving Trust, which helps us let go and trust others with tiny tasks. This practice can help you, much like it helped my client Yara trust her friend with concert tickets, to increase your trust gradually by first visualizing trust and pairing it with a relaxation practice called Progressive Muscle Relaxation. This will require that you sit in a comfortable seat, as you will be intentionally tensing up certain muscle groups in order to release the stress-based tension they are holding. Let's get started.

- Find a comfortable seat, preferably in your designated safe space.
- Find your breath and deepen it by increasing the inhale and exhale.
- Take three additional deep, slow breaths.
- And when you're ready, close your eyes.
- Envision a vulnerability that you have, a very small vulnerability, not something deeply vulnerable like fear of abandonment, but smaller, like a fear of heights.
- See yourself holding that vulnerability in your hand, as if it were an object.

- Envision someone who you already feel is a safe person to you, but who doesn't know about this vulnerability.
- Now envision that person's palms opening up to receive the gift of your vulnerability.
- When you're ready, envision yourself giving it over to that person.
- Notice how it feels to give them this gift of trust.
- What emotions come up for you?
- How connected are you feeling to them in this moment?
- Now shift your focus to your body.
- Start with your head and face. Are there any sensations you notice here?
- Take a deep breath in and scrunch up your face like you just ate something sour.
- Release your breath, release your facial tension, and notice any sensations it leaves behind.
- Now envision this person holding on to your trust in their hands for a few moments.
- As you do, shift your body focus to your heart.
- Breathe in a deep breath and give yourself a really tight hug.
- Release the hug, release your breath, and notice the sensations it leaves behind.
- Now envision this person holding your trust in their hands, caring for it and nurturing it.
- Breathe in a deep breath; squeeze the muscles in your core.
- Now release the muscles, release the breath, and notice the sensations it leaves behind.
- Now think of that person telling you, "You can trust me with this."
- Breathe in a deep breath; tense the muscles in your legs by squeezing them together.
- Release the muscles, release the breath, and notice what you feel.
- Now imagine yourself receiving your trust back, placed safely in your hands.

- Breathe in a deep breath and scrunch up your fingers and toes.
- Release them, release the breath, and notice the sensations.
- Sit here for a moment.
- Notice the way your body feels and the abundant releasing and receiving it just experienced.
- Take as many breaths as you need here.
- And when you're ready, open your eyes.

It always helps to write about our experiences. So if you're willing, take out your journal and write about what it was like to hand over trust to someone in this visualization practice. Did you notice any resistance coming up? What do you believe that resistance was keeping you from experiencing? And how might that resistance be a key to unlocking new generational insights about yourself?

Remember that reprogramming our nervous system takes hundreds of repetitions, so be sure to come back and do this practice as many times as needed. What we are doing here is training your intergenerational nervous system to expand its own limitations with regard to relationships and help your body absorb that it is safe to do so.

What You've Learned So Far

This chapter highlighted ways in which you have been a recipient of intergenerational resilience and the ways in which you can continue to build upon your strengths through an intergenerational post-traumatic growth process. You were guided through an exercise on building trust, helping you tune in to your own relaxation response and expand your intergenerational window of tolerance to foster deeper connections. Here, you were also offered multiple moments of reflection, so if it helps, take a gentle pause before diving into our final chapter on leaving a generational legacy.

REFLECTION QUESTIONS

How was it for you to learn about all of these layers of
   intergenerational resilience and growth?
What's one way you can remind yourself of your intergenerational
   strength each day?
In what other ways are you hoping to honor the ancestral resilience
   that lives in you?

CHAPTER 12

Leaving a Generational Legacy

I am not just my ancestors' wildest dreams.
I am my descendants' greatest hope.

—Unknown

You are the alchemist of your family's intergenerational legacy. Within this book, you have been creating the building blocks of that inheritance of healing, one that will impact you, your family, and your communities. Every chapter you've read, every skill you've learned, and every breath you've taken have drawn you closer to your legacy. As you've taken these steps to heal yourself, you've offered healing to your lineage and created an abundant foundation for generations to come.

A legacy is an opportunity to live in alignment with a bigger purpose; that purpose here is one of breaking the cycle of trauma. It's about living a less passive life that asserts only that you are the product of intergenerational trauma and living a more active life where you take steps toward creating a new narrative for yourself and your lineage. Generations after you will know what you've done here. They will tell stories about how you disrupted family patterns, how you advocated for your communities, and how you shifted history. You will be an ancestor that's spoken of because of the courage you've taken to step out of the status quo. Your newly acquired knowledge, your actions, and your wisdom will be recycled, time and again, generation after generation. That's the consequence of legacy building. It is the setup to have generational impact that transcends your life.

Through your cycle-breaking work, you have been obtaining generational privilege for yourself and anyone connected to you. Generational privilege is the privilege of knowledge, meaning knowing that intergenerational trauma exists, and the privilege of doing better, meaning choosing to create a new legacy. Intergenerational healing itself is a privilege. It offers you the *choice* to break the cycle. Because when you don't know that you are in a lineage of trauma, or have the tools to break out of it, you are more likely to stay in cycles. When you are offered a choice and the tools to disrupt, you gain generational privilege. So by doing this work, by learning how to heal, by choosing to obstruct trauma, you are using that generational privilege to become a legacy-building ancestor. You are becoming the ancestor you needed and the ancestor whom others will take pride in.

Becoming the Ancestor You Needed

Becoming a legacy-building ancestor will require you to embody your own healing and be dedicated to leaving behind some wisdom for others to carry. Embodying that intergenerational ancestral self that you learned about in chapter 2 is a selfless position. It means that you heal for yourself but also for the collective. It's about understanding that your healing is necessary so that your life can be filled with greater peace, but also so that you don't pass on a hurt-filled fate to future generations. I remember the first moment I thought of myself as a living ancestor. I was asked the question by my dear friend Layla Saad, "How does one become a good ancestor?" I remember responding by saying, "By looking back to the people that held on to hope. We won't solve everything in our lifetime. Any little bit that you can deposit into this world to make it a place where we can exist in our collective humanity, do it. Hold yourself accountable for that part . . . and let the world do the rest." I still hold the same position. We each do our part. We each break cycles and those actions, taken together, create a generational shift that will impact our collective descendants. We don't each have to change the entire world alone; we simply do our part. So what will your part be? What's your legacy? What change will you hold yourself responsible for? These questions may feel big and existential, but I can assure you that you are already doing a lot of what is asked here. I am simply asking you to reflect on it and act on it with intention. You can choose to take this moment to journal about your legacy. If you do so, here are some additional prompts you can consider as you write:

- What was the legacy you were left with?
- What would you like to keep from that legacy?
- What are you hoping to discard from it?
- What are some of the cultural values you're hoping to transition forward?
- What cultural values are you willing to discard?
- What behaviors are reflective of your intergenerational higher self?
- What behaviors are not?
- What stories will people tell about you in future generations?

You have been chosen for this task. The task of shifting. The task of disrupting the narrative that says, "This is as good as it gets," and shifting to a narrative that asserts that "it only gets better from here." You're generating an inheritance that's driven by a daily lived practice of showing up as your intergenerational higher self. It's in the daily commitment to heal back, heal laterally, and heal forward. To rise from the ashes of who you once were. To step into your power. The power of cycle breakers is the power to build intergenerational legacies. So take this moment to gather what that legacy will truly look like. Your ancestors have been waiting with anticipation for you to find yourself here, breaking cycles that honor both you and them. What would they say about how you're creating a legacy? How can you make them and yourself proud? And how will you help your descendants feel the same?

Cycle-Breaking Parenting

Some of us in this generation have made the decision to not have children as a way to discontinue the transmission of trauma-based genetic expressions, behaviors, and intergenerational ACEs that have run rampant in our lineage for generations. This can also be your version of giving the gift of ease to your lineage and making yourself and your ancestors proud. However, if you have decided that a part of your legacy is to parent in a way that also breaks the cycle, it will be critical for you to also have a road map for what cycle-breaking parenting can look like. Remember the concept of breaking parenting cycles we discussed in chapter 7? Well, let's take a moment to explore this concept further.

For some cycle breakers, the idea of creating a legacy of prosperity means that they teach future generations how to live differently than how they were taught by their own caregivers. Someone who chooses to parent as a cycle breaker is stepping up to a big challenge. They are mostly enacting new parenting practices out of sheer intuition and attempting to build a different foundation for their children and the generations that follow them. Some clients who I have worked with care deeply about future generations but are not yet parents. One of my clients didn't have kids but knew she wanted them someday. She once called herself a *preemptive cycle breaker*, because she was doing the work of self-regulation, giving herself the chance to be as grounded and healed as she could be, before her children were even conceived. If you're there, or if you're a parent already, thinking about the parental impact you can have is a healthy legacy-building practice.

Many cycle breakers who grew up with intergenerational ACEs tend to worry about what kind of parent they will be and about passing on generational cycles to their children. Parents worry about the possibility of fractured attachments, rejection, shame, and oppression, among other things. They want to parent differently, because they wish they were parented differently. They want to live in a world that feels safer, because they grew up in a world where consistent safety didn't exist. They don't want their children to be inheritors of traumatized minds, bodies, and genes. Oftentimes, it's this dedication that cycle breakers have to their children that functions as the greatest motivator to break cycles. I hear so many parent clients say, "All I know is I don't want to do things like my mother. I want to do things differently for my child." For many parents, their cycle-breaking process stems from feelings that are rooted in their own inner child desires. It's from that revelation of wanting a different inner child experience for their own kids that cycle breakers find intuitive ways to shift the generational narrative. They look at the patterns reflected in their Intergenerational Trauma Tree and want to create new leaves with more adaptive and healthy patterns, rather than the destructive ones that they have seen represented down their family line. One client, when she experienced a fork in the road in her parenting, would often ask herself, "What would I have wanted my parent to do in this situation?" And in those moments, she would offer herself an opportunity to think reflectively about what her next step would be. This reflection can also be a healthy pause you can initiate in your own parenting. I find that it grounds parents and aligns with their desire for their children's lives to feel different from their own childhoods. Some common wishes I have heard other parents relay to me over the years have been:

- "It is important to not raise my child in fear, in the ways that I was raised."
- "I want to be able to have open communication with my child about their expected behavior without resorting to physical harm in order to get my point across."
- "I want my child to feel like they matter to me and that they matter in general."
- "I didn't feel like I had a voice in my home growing up. I want my child to feel heard and seen."
- "My child has a lot of energy like I had at their age. I was punished so much for it. I want them to feel like their energy isn't wrong or bad, but something to be celebrated."
- "I want my child to feel proud about who they are."
- "I want my child to feel like they can play and not have to worry about their childhood being taken away."
- "I want my child to learn what to keep and what to discard when it comes to cultural values."
- "I want my child to feel like they can openly express their emotions without me suppressing or invalidating them. That was very much the norm in my home back in the day."
- "I want my child to hear me say 'I'm sorry' when I make a mistake and know that they are worthy of an apology."
- "I want my child to have a childhood that feels happy, supported, and safe."
- "I want my child to feel empowered to make changes in the world for their children and their children's children."

The good news is that, as you've learned throughout this book, a legacy of trauma can be redirected. Parents who suffered trauma in their childhood can safeguard their children from the damaging experiences they had to suffer. Even if their children are born with emotional vulnerabilities already, exposing them to different parenting practices can help strengthen their resilience and help them lead lives filled with ease.

Breaking Old Parenting Patterns

Parenting from a cycle-breaking lens integrates two complementary practices: caring for yourself and caring for your children. When parents have improved emotion regulation skills, they're able to be more mindful of their parenting practices and create healthier communication with their kids. Enhanced parental mindfulness facilitates, for parents, a better understanding of their own needs and their children's needs simultaneously, which boosts their capacity for attunement. This means that as a cycle-breaking parent, you will have to continuously provide attunement and regulation to your children (caring for them), while providing attunement to yourself (caring for yourself). You will also need to create a psychologically safe environment for your children (caring for them), while still learning what psychological safety even is (caring for yourself). If you're a parent, you'll have to work twice as hard at breaking cycles. Despite it not being an easy task, for many parents it is a worthwhile one.

When parents ask me, "How do I ensure that I'm not passing intergenerational trauma on to my child?" I recommend they start by settling their *own* mind, body, and spirit to ensure that their child has a safer home to return to. Remember Luna and how she and I first worked on settling her nervous system so that she could truly see her child's needs? That's the type of work that will also be necessary for you to do. By focusing on settling your nervous system, you can better ensure that your child is not returning to a home that's filled with emotional chaos, but is instead able to feel seen. You are ensuring that their legacy isn't one that reflects a chaotic childhood, but one marked by emotional stability.

Typically, when a child comes in for therapy, a large part of the work is done with the parents. We train the adults on how to adjust their parenting technique so that the child's behavior can start shifting in the direction of health. If as a parent you're unconsciously engaging in trauma responses, you can risk creating an imbalance in your child's nervous system and perpetuating the inherited trauma cycle. Alternatively, your capacity to step out of that reactive behavior cycle and understand your child's needs is a useful inhibitor of the transmission of intergenerational trauma. That is why the work with parents is so important when considering the impact on children.

The way that I work with parent cycle breakers is through a process I call Parenting Back–Parenting Forward. It's a process that honors the parents' emotional world, as well as their child's. It's a way to help you adopt a more mindful approach to parenting that considers the different layers of intergenerational healing.

The first part of this process is Parenting Back, or intergenerational reparenting. You focus on giving yourself what your intergenerational inner child needs. This means settling your intergenerational nervous system in the ways you learned in chapter 6, doing the intergenerational inner child work we discussed in chapter 7, and working on creating a more grounded mind, body, and spirit for yourself each day. This will allow you an opportunity to feel cared for and more settled. The added bonus is that you can develop a greater emotional attunement to your own needs, so that you can show up as a more emotionally mature and emotionally stable parent.

As you can see, this is the stuff you've been learning, so you are already setting up the work for the second part of this process, Parenting Forward. That is the commitment you can make to consciously focus on legacy-centered parenting each day, meaning the parenting that helps you stay mindful of your generational impact on your children. This way, you can pause and reflect on how you could either be keeping cycles or creating legacies and make a *choice* on which direction you are willing to take. Some Parenting Forward considerations include:

- **Regulate Their Nervous System**—Teach your children how to regulate their nervous systems early so that they can have a better biological foundation than you had. This can start as early as before conception, when they're in the womb, or birth. However, it's never too late to learn a skill that can help with managing stress, so no matter the age of your child, think about introducing them to deep breathing, meditation, or even dance parties that can help them better absorb stress. Coregulating with children teaches them the art of finding peace. Humming, rocking, and other nervous system exercises can be a set of default practices that they can always turn to when life gets rough.

- **Help Them Form a Secure Attachment**—As you've learned through these pages and probably even know from your own experiences, parental emotional attunement is critical to develop a secure attachment. So, it will be important to become more emotionally available to your children than your parents were in your infancy. This is not about achieving perfection and being 100 percent attentive, but rather it's about scaling it up. It's about looking into your child's eyes, like Luna did, and noticing their emotional and physical needs. If this feels like a hard task for you to simply do out of intuition and if your child has verbal capacities, you can try asking your child, "What can I offer you right now?" and do your best to provide that. Helping children cultivate attachment security by helping them see that a parent is consistently present, caring, and loving is essential.

- **Model Safety for Them**—Help your children see you as their safe person. We first learn about psychological safety in our homes. If your children are able to establish a safe base with their caregivers, they can go out into the world with less fear and doubt.

- **Affirm Your Child**—Affirming a child can help them build the language that they will then internalize about themselves. You can help them develop this internal language by first affirming them with the words that pierce their soul. Tell them what you wish them to hear. If it helps, you can simply start with "I see you," "I hear you," "I value you." These affirmations will help them feel seen, heard, and valued, which will later translate into them seeing, hearing, and valuing themselves.

- **Don't Hit Your Child**—Physical punishment sends children down a psychological spiral and teaches them negative messages about their bodies being a recipient of retribution. When a child feels they are in danger, their cortical brain, which they need for higher-level understanding, temporarily slows down, and they can't adequately process whatever it is you need them to do. Hitting a child can place them in survival mode, and from that place they won't be able to fully comprehend your instructions. Instead, consider alternate ways of relaying the messages you wish them to hear. This is where a settled intergenerational nervous system also comes into play, because it allows you to communicate more effectively and give them an instruction that they can hear more clearly.

- **Prioritize Their Voice and Opinion**—Increasing your child's independence and agency makes a difference in how they evolve. Children in households with intergenerational trauma feel like they lack a voice in their home. Breaking that cycle means making a child's voice prominent and heard. This will also help them go out into the world with confidence and not shrink themselves.

- **Let Them Tell You How They Feel**—Helping your children adequately express how they feel is so powerful. If we teach children how to feel their emotions safely early on, they won't have to be the adults in search of a healthy expression of their emotions later in life, meaning that they won't have to spend years of their lives reconnecting to their authentic expressions of emotions because they never learned how to sit with their own feelings. Creating a childhood centered on the full expression of their feelings helps safeguard your children from having to spend years on inner child healing when they're older.

- **Apologize to Your Children**—Apologies are a sign of courage and compassion. You can offer your child an apology and in turn reflect to them that their emotions matter. You can also help them learn to apologize for a misstep by modeling this for them. It is a way in which you can both be flawed humans who see each other fully, like a *true* family would, and allow room for errors and repair.

- **Let Them Get Creative**—Helping children foster creative expression is key. Generational cycles stunt creativity, so it's essential to help them garner the freedom to expand. Allowing them to do so is a way you can also stretch your own creativity, especially if it was stunted by a traumatic upbringing.

- **Let Them Play**—It's so important that we allow children to play. So many people across the world are trying to get back to their inner child through play, because they didn't get enough opportunities to enjoy their leisure time back when they were kids. But maybe if we allow children to jump in puddles, laugh out loud, go on swings, roll down hills, and do kids' stuff, they won't desperately search for these experiences as adults.

- **Vet the People You Leave Your Children With**—Vetting the people we leave our children with can help safeguard them more. It is OK to ask your children's caretakers about how they will protect your child and confirm that they will not violate them. It's a taboo topic, but like many topics we keep in the shadows, we won't be able to resolve it until we shed light on it and have courageous conversations about this difficult subject. It can be the conversation that can help keep your child safe.

- **Believe Your Children**—In addition to vetting who is around them, you must also make it a practice to talk to your children about their own body boundaries. It is critical to always leave room to talk to children about any people whom they have contact with and believe your children if they tell you that someone has hurt them. It's important in these moments for you to settle your nervous system so that you can respond to your children in the most child-centered way, where they feel heard and protected, not shamed and retraumatized.

- **Balance Their Worldview**—It's critical to teach children to scan the world for positive attributes. Remember that trauma preprograms a person to search for threats and can keep them stuck in hypervigilance. Focusing on positive attributes can help balance the lens through which they see the world, so that they understand that there are dangers in the world but that there are also wonderful things about it.

- **Teach Them to Understand Their Impact**—You can teach your children to be community-centered in life and to care for the life and humanity of others. Teach them this, because our humanity depends upon each other and because their capacity to stay well will always be connected to the wellness of their community. Imagine if we, as a generation of cycle breakers, commit to teaching the next generation this concept. The generation that follows can be even more interdependent and conscious of their collective impact. Yes, this is possible, and each of us can do our part.

- **Advocate for a World That Doesn't Rob Them of Their Childhood**—Go out into the world and develop change that can keep your child safer and more joyful. Advocate for safety laws, practices, and values that can shield your child from intergenerational adverse experiences, particularly those that happen on the collective level and later pour into their home.

- **Let Them Gather Wisdom**—Consider expanding your children's interactions with other people in the community. Have them talk to elders and community veterans to gain generational wisdom and wealth outside their home and school environments.

How Do I Know My Child Is OK?

As a cycle-breaking parent, you may be harboring a valid concern about whether your child has already been an inheritor of intergenerational trauma. It's common for parents to worry and have looping thoughts like, "Did I pass it on?" "Am I doing this right?" "How do I know I haven't messed them up?" and "If I did, how do I make it right?" Frankly, living in this ongoing state of worry is not going to help you focus on your child's needs. Quite the opposite actually, because a worried mind is not an attuned mind.

It's natural to feel some sense of helplessness in your cycle-breaking parenting journey. You are doing hard work. However, refocusing that anxious energy into helping your child feel more regulated can offer you a better chance at helping them than staying anxious ever will. These are excellent moments to parent back and give yourself what you need so that you can more effectively parent forward. You can buffer the possibility of inflicting trauma by first modeling how you are taking better care of yourself, then by talking to your children about their needs.

In Japan, there's a saying that children learn by watching what their parents do, not by hearing what they say. A child observes how their parent employs self-care and often mirrors that in their own burgeoning personality. When we model care and calmer nervous systems for children, they feel emboldened by it, mimic it, and become calm themselves. They start to embody the legacy you are creating.

I once worked with the family of an adolescent child who was my "identified patient," meaning they were the person the family came to me to "fix." Some weeks into our work together, while having session with both the parents and the child, I realized that the entire family was experiencing a collective emotional chaos. Their intergenerational nervous systems were inflamed and firing against each other. We had to engage in Parenting Back–Parenting Forward regulation practices in order to reestablish the parent-child attachment processes.

Some of our practices were family ventral vagal toning, which was especially helpful to their teenager, who struggled with regulating their emotions on a daily basis and who especially benefited from emotion regulation in session. The entire family would hum the same Spanish song that they would sing to their children when they were little. Those moments were heartwarming to watch, because they were collectively healing, but also because the teenager would have a really positive response to the practice. But my absolute favorite moments with the family were when we would all do dance movement therapy together. Not only was it helping their intergenerational nervous systems regulate through the practice itself, but oftentimes the teenager would giggle at some of the moves, which would make the parents start laughing. And I understood in that moment that so much was happening generationally; their mirror neurons were syncing to laughter, their nervous systems were registering a collective relaxation response, and they were sharing a beautiful moment of intergenerational coregulation together. A large part of why this regulation needed to be done within their cycle-breaking parenting was because their hurt was intertwined, so we needed to intertwine their healing. You, too, can interconnect your healing with your children's healing and create legacies together through the practices reflected here.

My client Yara wanted to parent differently. You may remember the story of when Yara's dad forgot to pick her up from school. That was traumatic for Yara, and so the way she engaged in her own Parenting

Back–Parenting Forward practices was by giving herself the affirmations she needed to internalize that she didn't deserve to be abandoned. Parenting Forward for Yara consisted of showing up at every school pickup for her own children. Yara even went further to tell her kids how much she loved being present for them and how valuable they were to her. This allowed them to understand that even if she were to miss a pickup, she was present and devoted to their wellness and safety. These actions instilled parental pride in Yara. She parented differently because she wanted to relay a different message to her kids: "I am here, I am consistent, and it is an honor for me to show up for you." It's a vastly different message from what she internalized in her own childhood: that she wasn't valuable and that she was a burden to her parents. She learned to parent back and parent forward so that she could break the cycle for her children while she continued to break the cycle within herself.

Stepping Into Our Legacies

These days, my mom still keeps a garage full of *stuff*, things she planned to one day send home to the DR. My preprogrammed response to seeing these items has always been to mentally shut down and numb my emotions. I would slump and feel a wave of exhaustion take over my body. I felt the guilt and grief held in those unshipped boxes. It was all-consuming.

My response now is to breathe. I remember when I reacted this way for the first time. I laughed and said, "Oh my goodness, I just took a deep breath subconsciously." My body did the healing by default. It was beautiful. I felt lighter. I didn't shut down. I didn't fight. I safely stayed there and noticed that I was in a body of ease. I was in generational flow, and not in generational constriction. I knew how significant that one automatic deep breath was. I had adopted a new default behavior.

It had taken hundreds of repetitions. But here I was, living in the embodiment of a more regulated nervous system, feeling closer to my intergenerational higher self, and seeing the legacy of all the work I had done.

I felt calm and deeply proud, but my work has not stopped there. My family continues to have ongoing conversations about our healing. We continue to engage in daily self-care practices, both together and on our own. We tell each other generational stories of pain and triumph, leaving space for vulnerability with one another. We excavate the skeletons in our closet and do so with compassion. We are modeling this to my nephew and creating a new foundation for him. That's a legacy we are collectively proud of.

My clients Nola, Yara, Brooklyn, Leon, Zuri, Solomon, Luna, and countless others have each disrupted their cycles and built new legacies with cycle breaking at the center. The work that we did together, minute by minute, session by session, has also made me proud.

I'm also profoundly proud of you and the work you've done along this journey. This is a journey of unbecoming and unlearning. It's a journey of reestablishing the person you are beyond the layers of trauma. It's one of showing up in a regulated nervous system more often than not. And when you do, seeing it as a part of how you're living in the intergenerational legacy that you have created. That's something that I hope can also make you eternally proud.

Breaking the Cycle: Alchemizing Your Legacy

In the Dominican Republic, the government turns off all electricity and gas sporadically throughout the week. You'll hear people yelling from their homes to their neighbors, "Se fue la luz!" ("The lights went out!") This means that whatever was in the refrigerator and is perishable will go to waste. But the resourceful people of the DR found ways to come together during these almost daily disruptions. Neighbors take any perishable foods and create meals to feed each other when the lights go out. Traditionally, they make sancocho, a stew of root vegetables and all the meats that are in the fridge. When my family would make sancocho, it would be in the dark, in our backyard, over fire (a very old and ancient practice). The stew is made in a huge pot that measures about two feet in diameter. And it feeds anyone who's near: family, friends, neighbors, anyone.

My paternal grandmother, Mamá María, taught her children, including my dad, how to make a sancocho. I hear she would always save a plate for whoever needed an extra meal in the neighborhood: el pasajero, she would call them, meaning whoever *passes by* the home. I learned a lesson about alchemy when I saw my dad making the sancocho his mother used to make and feeding anyone who was hungry. Our whole family contributed to helping my dad prepare the ingredients for the feast. One person washed the meats, another person peeled the vegetables, and another gathered the wood for the fire. Everyone combined efforts to create this massively nourishing meal in the dark. And it reminds me of what we're doing here with this work; we are cooking in the darkness of our pain, throwing in everything that we want to salvage into the healing pot and leaving a little extra for anyone else who needs some healing too. As a final exercise, I wanted to make a metaphorical sancocho with you.

- Take a piece of paper and draw a circle to signify the pot.
- Now draw the ingredients (potato, plantains, yuca, chicken, smoked beef, pork sausage, corn, and dumplings).
- Above each of the ingredients, write what you are adding to your sancocho (everything you wish to salvage from this journey, like daily practices that create generational strength, the practice of apologizing to your children, the practice of writing letters to your ancestors, etc.).

- Now draw the fire beneath the pot. The fire signifies what will keep the sancocho cooking but also what will keep you fired up as you're building this legacy.
- Write a few words on the fire that signify what will keep you motivated.
- Now take this sancocho drawing and any of your other items and practices you have collected along this journey.
- Place them all in a container with your journal.
- Anytime that you need reminders, skills, or practice, you can go back into your container and grab what you need.

What You've Learned So Far

In this chapter, you more concretely focused on how you can build and sustain an intergenerational legacy. You learned ways to parent from an intergenerational parenting model, Parenting Back–Parenting Forward, and to use specific tools to deepen growth and abundance in your healing journey. You were also prompted to create a legacy sancocho to identify what you'll be keeping as a part of your intergenerational legacy journey. Dive into your reflection questions before heading to some final words I have for you to carry with you.

REFLECTION QUESTIONS

How has your learning about generational legacy building changed how you see your generational healing journey?

What are your thoughts on intergenerational reparenting, caring for yourself while caring for the next generation?

How are you hoping your journey could impact future generations?

How are you hoping to carry this work forward?

EPILOGUE

This book was cultivated out of a deep desire to see a generational shift in how we approach trauma healing. I knew I wanted people to experience profound healing in the pages of this book, but once it was time to write the words, I was stuck on how to write it. I asked my sister, Lady, "How will I write an entire book that reflects a decade of therapeutic work and generations of stories? I don't even know where to start." She responded by saying, "Just write the book you needed." This is that book. It's the book I needed in my own intergenerational healing. It's the book that reflects how countless others have also healed. It's the book that grew out of alchemized lessons of generational wisdom from my therapy room. This book reflects my clients' courage and trust. It's a book that reflects my ancestors' wisdom. It demonstrates my family's strength. And it reveals my love for healing people's souls. For healing yours.

This book was made for you, for us. For the brave. For those who want to step into courage and heal. Throughout this book, I wanted to reflect tested and true therapeutic practices but also, and perhaps most importantly, the voices of cycle breakers. I wanted to elevate and feature the voices of the generation who chose to break the cycle. As a fellow cycle breaker, I wanted your experiences to be reflected here too.

I wanted you to feel seen in the pages of this book and for you to feel less alone in this courageous journey. I hope that as you have read each word, you have felt this; you have felt seen, fully.

I created this book with profound intention. I wanted to equip you with an abundance of knowledge to help empower you, which is why I made sure to cover the science behind this healing protocol. I also wanted you to not just learn about intergenerational healing but to have a guide to put it into practice. This book serves as that road map toward healing lineage trauma.

In the first part of this book, "What You Inherited," I wanted you to start seeing how you got into the cycle of generational pain, but more importantly, I wanted you to see that you also came equipped to do this work. You were able to adopt your own unique cycle-breaker identity while breaking up with the identity that had trauma at the center. This was a critical step in your evolution and healing, so it was an important foundation to lay in your journey. You then transitioned into acknowledging and stepping into more of the generational resilience that exists in you. Our generational resilience is oftentimes overlooked, and so it was that much more important to help you not only remember that it's there but absorb that wisdom in a more profound way. We then focused on the body, which is necessary to do when we want to transition out of survival mode.

You were able to capture how the body is impacted both in the short term and long term by the chronic stress connected to trauma. You then learned how to achieve deep, ancestral relaxation of your nervous system through your Breaking the Cycle practice. But also, you learned how critical it is to integrate this deep nervous system reset into your daily life, in order to offset the impact of generations of trauma. Then, you learned about the layers of trauma and both the biological and psychological remnants of this type of emotional injury. This is where you started the intergenerational mapping of your wounds through the development of your Intergenerational Trauma Healing Assessment and your Intergenerational Trauma Tree, which helped you understand what happened to you, through the generations. You did some heavy lifting here and added language and tools to your intergenerational toolbox that were an essential first step toward your emotional liberation.

In the second part, "There Are Layers to This," I purposefully started adding layers to your learning. Each of these was an important piece of the puzzle that I wanted you to acquire and was critical in helping you understand the full landscape of intergenerational trauma.

You were able to capture the intergenerational threads of triggers, memories, and of your nervous system, while learning how to release those traumatic memories from your soul. You were also able to dive into one of the hardest concepts for cycle breakers to internalize about generational pain, which is the fact that our parents can have unresolved inner child wounds that get passed on generationally. This realization comes with a lot of mixed emotions about the pain they could have caused by not resolving their own wounds, but it also comes with an opportunity to heal what they couldn't. In order to do that work, it was critical for you to map out a more extensive intergenerational adverse childhood experience that answered the questions "What happened to you?" "What happened before you?" and "What happened around you?" And because we don't exist in isolation, but in cultures that breed trauma, it was critical for you to capture how cycles of abuse, toxicity, harmful cultural values, and systemic diseases are also a part of this massive web of intergenerational trauma. Through it all, you were called to do something about these layers of trauma. You were guided on how to abandon inaction and act at the individual and collective level, so your own liberation from intergenerational trauma can be more sustainable.

And finally, in part 3, "Alchemizing Your Legacy," we shed the old and invited in abundance. Your intergenerational post-traumatic growth was central in this section, and you needed to shed the layers of pain, expectations, and values that no longer serve you. This was a moment of grief and loss but also of elevation and evolution. Here, we increased your capacity for resilience, which transcends generations, while also looking out for future generations through parenting approaches that center your intergenerational goal of abundance. And finally, we ended with building your legacy and concretizing what your new inheritance will reflect, for yourself and for the generations to come. This was the setup for the rest of your life, a life of intergenerational liberation.

Now, you're here, having gone through the full healing protocol. This is the moment when you get to shake that family tree and allow the last set of rotting leaves to fall. This is the moment when you trim the roots that have been growing your pain and change that barren soil. In this era of your life, your tree's trunk will grow new rings that reflect how you broke the cycle. In nature, when an event happens that changes the tree's environment, like a major storm or an earthquake, it leaves a mark on the tree's growth rings that indicates that a major shift has happened. When you break the cycle of trauma, you leave a similar imprint in the trunk of your family tree. You leave a mark that signifies that a major shift has happened. What's also beautiful about this process is that a tree's old rings become known as the dead part of the tree, and the new rings mark what keeps the tree alive. So the growth you create out of your cycle-breaking era will be what keeps you and your lineage alive and abundant. You have done that, through your courage. Building a generational legacy is possible, and it starts with the one soul who finds the courage to do so. You are that person. You are the ancestor of your descendants' wildest dreams. You are the hero of your lineage.

Intergenerational healing work requires your daily commitment to step into courage in the ways you have done throughout this book. The rest of the journey ahead will be made up of small moments that continue to build upon the legacy you have formulated here. It will require that you commit to leaving old patterns behind, that you shed the identity and personality that made you a cycle keeper, and that you continue to release yourself from both people and norms that breed trauma. It will be a journey where you place ancestral rest at the center, because honoring your own healing helps your ancestors rest easy, because they understand that you're doing the hard work of helping liberate your lineage from burdens. This is where you commit to not stepping back into the cycle and even to connecting with people who are equally committed to the same. When you shed the old, you welcome in a space to replace it with something that will embody abundance. So as a final reflection question for you, I ask, "What will take the place of those old patterns?" You get to choose. You have a choice. That is a source of empowerment that no trauma can take away from you. And the added beauty of it is, you get to make this choice every single day. Each day, you will be presented with new opportunities to continue breaking cycles. I hope that you choose the path of courage and come back to any of the practices that feel necessary to continue building your generational health.

My mother recently uttered some beautiful words to my father, my sister, and me that helped me understand more fully what this cycle-breaking journey urges us to do. In reflecting on all that she has suffered, and all the pain that others have caused her, she said she was no longer willingly holding on to pain. At the age of sixty-five, she committed to letting go of the weight she had carried around for over six decades. She put the baggage down. She no longer wanted to load her back with the intergenerational guilt she had carried in the luggage she transported from the Dominican Republic. She was ready to step into intergenerational abundance. In doing so, she said the most heal-centered words I have ever heard my mother say. She said, "Estoy en mi era de paz." ("I am in my peace era.") My mother is living out her legacy of peace, and I'm getting to witness her laugh like her inner child never had a chance to and hug us without overburdening emotions overtaking her, and I get to see her eyes reflect unhindered joy. My father also expressed a thought that tugged at my heart and helped me see the abundance that we have been living in. He and I were having a heartfelt conversation about the generations of our family and the one core aspect that has kept our family rooted, despite the multiple ways in which our lives have been pummeled by pain. He noted that regardless of how much we have each endured, we continue to pass on an "inheritance of love." That is the legacy that my parents have been able to offer me. A legacy of love. Love in action. I have taken that and grieved what they could not provide. I took what they offered me and created love in the form of healing, here, for all of us to always fall back onto, in the very ways I fall back into my parents' arms for love. My mom and dad have evolved so much in their healing, as has my sister, as have I. My nephew, Aiden, the legacy bearer, gets to experience a family that is deep in generational freedom, rather than deep in generational trauma. And I can't think of a better gift to offer our dear descendant, in his generation.

My clients and family both have been the guides to helping make this book a powerful healing tool for a whole generation of cycle breakers and legacy builders. I hope you have been able to see how this book is your companion in building that legacy for you, as it has been for all of us. I hope this becomes the book you needed, the one you waited for, the one that helped you heal, and the book that you feel you can nestle back into time and again. Come back to it as often as you need. Share it with people who may need to heal. And let's continue to disrupt harmful imprints for generations to come.

Acknowledgments

First and foremost, thank you to my family, for giving space to our ongoing healing and for your willingness to allow our story to be reflected on the pages of this book, for others to also heal with.

I would also like to extend a warm thank-you to:

My editors, Cassidy Sachs and Sam Jackson, for your incredible guidance and gentle care with every word reflected in this healing guide. Cassidy, you are simply the best thought partner I could have asked for. Your gentle approach to my work both helped me get through the arduous parts of writing and stretched me beyond any capacity I thought I possessed as an author. Thank you for putting so much into this title and pouring into me. I appreciate you more than you know. Sam, you have been a necessary voice and balance in this book. You have helped me to understand how to zoom in and out of my work in ways that were so necessary—a skill I will always carry with me. Thank you both so much for what you have deposited into this book. I'm so proud of what we've created here.

My brilliant agents, Katherine Latshaw and Sonali Chanchani, for believing in this book and in its mission to build a generation of cycle breakers. Katherine, since the first day we met, I have sensed your heartfelt commitment not only to this book, but to helping me establish my own voice as an author. And you do it all with so much humor and lightheartedness. It's one of my favorite qualities about you, among all the things there are to love. Sonali, your ability to hold this vision of mine with such meticulous care is unmatched. Your devotion is something that I feel each time we connect and I'm so honored that you are helping me to bring this title into the world. You have carried both me and this project with so much grace and I'm so grateful for that and for you.

To every team member at Dutton who has so graciously offered their expertise and contributed to the making of *Break the Cycle*—including Stephanie Cooper, Diamond Bridges, Lauren Morrow, Hannah Poole, Amanda Walker, Marie Finamore, Heather Rodino, and everyone who has helped bring this book to life—thank you, truly.

My mentors, Dr. Diana Puñales-Morejón, Dr. Santos Vales, Dr. Traci Stein, Dr. Elizabeth Fraga, and Dr. Dinelia Rosa, who helped me find my clinical voice and step into this field with confidence and intention. Thank you for believing that my voice had a place in spaces where our voices aren't prominent. Thank you for helping me to believe the same. Santos and Diana, you filled a void in my world that can never again be emptied. Thank you for your love and care for me, familia. I love you dearly.

My sisters who have held space and care for me on this book journey. Dr. Courtney Rose, your sisterhood has been an invaluable part of my personal and professional growth and I am deeply grateful to know you and witness your genius throughout these years. Dr. Roshnee Vázquez, I'm so grateful for your support and believing in this book as much as you have, mil gracias mi hermana. Jodieann Nelson, my sister from another mother and such a champion of my work, your presence in my life is gold and I simply love growing old knowing you are a friend I can count on. My dearest Layla Saad, you are one of the most wholesome humans I know. I treasure you so much. Thank you for helping me to see myself as a living ancestor. And my sweet cousin Leezet Matos, you illuminate my life in so many ways. Thank you for just being the light that you are. Thank you for your sisterhood and keeping my thoughts and emotions as I navigated this book process.

The wonderful friends, and colleagues who have lifted my work and family, including Ana Flores, Vanessa Santos, Paula Duran, Aila Castane Jalloh, Melissa Bailey, María Fernanda Salaverría, Amy Morin, Lewis Howes, and Team Greatness, Dave Aizer, Kristie Usher, and Cookie Hopkins, thank you for your indispensable support, always.

To my extended family, Tía Nerys, Tivo, Chago, Tía Nini, Tía Piza, Tía Hilda, and mis hermanos, who have helped raise me and have nurtured and loved me always. Thank you for helping me become a woman of generational power and strength.

To the healers who have held space and care for me and for my family, Dr. Joseph Reynoso, Dr. Harish Seethamraju, Pam Philippsborn, Dr. Rajesh J. Pandey, Yolanda Amador, Alyssa Sandler, and Rocio Navarro. Thank you for your holistic and tailored care, on behalf of all of us.

To my little ones—Leo and Marley. Thank you for allowing me to pour love and care into your lives.

To Mamá, for being such a powerful force and guide in my life. I hope I have made you proud. Rest easy, mi vieja.

To my parents, Rammy and Margarita, thank you for your inheritance of love. But you gave me so much more than love. You gave me a strength that can only be explained as intergenerational. Your will to break cycles doesn't go unnoticed. I know you did your best. And I appreciate your best and have more love for you than my heart could possibly hold.

To my sister, Lady. My muse. My light. My life companion. We have lived every moment of life side by side. As Mom calls us, her right and left lungs, always breathing life into our family. Look at what we have birthed within this book. It is you who has created the will in me to help others heal. I hope you continue to always bloom and live in abundance. I will always be here with you to see that your life is filled with an overflow of love.

To Andy, my sweet little one. You are forever in my heart. Thank you for coming into our lives for those brief moments. We are forever better because of you.

To Aiden, my dear descendant, you are the center, the hub, the motivation for us all to be better humans. You amaze me every day of your life by simply being you. Always shine, always seek balance, and always know that you are loved.

To my clients. Thank you for honoring me with your stories and allowing me to carry your intergenerational histories alongside you. I hope you feel that I have carried them with care.

And to you, the cycle breakers of this world, thank you for the inspiration to create a healing protocol for us all. May you continue your legacy building, now and forever.

APPENDIX A

Mamá Tutúna's Lemongrass Healing Tea

Lemongrass has been known to boost immunity, help improve sleep, reduce pain, regulate sugar, regulate cholesterol levels, and regulate hormones, and it has antioxidant properties, among many other health-promoting benefits known for generations.

1 tablespoon chopped fresh lemongrass stalk
1 teaspoon grated fresh ginger
3 chopped fresh basil leaves
1 tablespoon honey
1 cinnamon stick

In a mug, combine the lemongrass, ginger, basil, honey, and cinnamon using a tea infuser. Add boiling water and let steep for 5 minutes before drinking.

Prep Time: 5 mindful minutes
Drink Time: 5 mindful minutes
Total Healing Time: 10 cycle-breaking minutes

Disclaimer on the Use of Herbs and Botanicals: Every person's body is made differently and will respond differently to natural herbs and botanicals. All recommendations proposed in this book are to be taken as informational only and used with caution. Please consult with local healers who are versed on the use of botanicals so that you can best learn what earthly medicine would make sense to introduce to your body, mind, and spirit.

APPENDIX B

Intergenerational Trauma Healing
Grounding Techniques

1. Emotional freedom technique (EFT)
2. Progressive muscle relaxation
3. Trauma-informed yoga
4. Lu Jong
5. Sound bath meditation
6. Ventral vagal nerve stimulation
7. Paced breathing
8. Guided meditation
9. Dance movement therapy
10. Imagery exercises
11. Body scans
12. Biofeedback
13. Rocking
14. Humming
15. Yoga nidra
16. Tai chi / qigong
17. Reciting mantras
18. Journaling
19. Stretching by candlelight
20. Grounding with the five senses

APPENDIX C

Holistic Healing Practices

1. Cupping therapy
2. Reflexology
3. Sauna treatments
4. Lymphatic massages
5. Nutritional supplementation
6. Acupuncture
7. Chakra balancing
8. Reiki
9. Mindful cooking and eating
10. Cold temperature stimulation
11. Balancing the gut flora
12. Aromatherapy
13. Horticulture (plant therapy)
14. Self-massages
15. Catching a sunrise or a sunset
16. Mindful walks outdoors
17. Hot baths
18. Tea ceremonies
19. Making art
20. Natural sunlight

APPENDIX D

Sound Bath Meditations

Scan to access sound baths curated by Dr. Mariel Buqué.

prh.com/marielbuquesoundbath

By scanning, I acknowledge that I have read and agree to Penguin Random House's Privacy Policy (prh.com/privacy) and Terms of Use (prh.com/terms) and understand that Penguin Random House collects certain categories of personal information for the purposes listed in that policy, discloses, sells, or shares certain personal information and retains personal information in accordance with the policy located here: prh.com/privacy. You can opt-out of the sale or sharing of personal information anytime from prh.com/privacy/right-to-opt-out-of-sale-form.

Bibliography

Chapter 1—You Are a Cycle Breaker

Duran, Eduardo. *Healing the Soul Wound: Trauma-Informed Counseling for Indigenous Communities.* New York: Teachers College Press, 2021.

Houck, James A. *When Ancestors Weep: Healing the Soul from Intergenerational Trauma.* Bloomington, IN: Abbott Press, 2018.

Chapter 2—Your Intergenerational Higher Self

Chopra, Deepak. *The Higher Self.* New York: Simon & Schuster, 2001.

Faddegon, Tom. "Using the Higher Self to Overcome False Beliefs." Higher Self Yoga, March 3, 2022. https://higherselfyoga.org/higher-self-overcome-false-beliefs.

Gaia staff. "How to Connect with the Divine Energy Your Higher Self Holds." Gaia, June 24, 2022. https://www.gaia.com/article/how-connect-your-divine-energy-self-4-steps.

Higher Self Yoga. "10 Ways to Connect with Your Higher Self." September 12, 2021. https://higherselfyoga.org/how-to-connect-with-your-higher-self.

John, Jaia. *Freedom: Medicine Words for Your Brave Revolution.* Camarillo, CA: Soul Water Rising, 2021.

Kaur, Rupi. *Home Body.* New York: Simon & Schuster, 2020.

Laz, Athena. "What Actually Is a 'Higher Self' & How Do I Connect to Mine?" *Mindbodygreen*, March 2, 2023. https://www.mindbodygreen.com/articles/connect-to-your-higher-self-what-this-phrase-really-means/.

Luna, Alethia. "Higher Self: 11 Ways to Connect with Your Soul." LonerWolf, October 27, 2022. https://lonerwolf.com/higher-self/.

O'Sullivan, Natalia, and Terry O'Sullivan. *Ancestral Healing Made Easy: How to Resolve Ancestral Patterns and Honour Your Family History.* London: Hay House, 2021.

Rogers, Scott L. *The Elements of Mindfulness: An Invitation to Explore the Nature of Waking Up to the Present Moment and Staying Awake.* New York: Mindful Living Press, 2017.

Yugay, Irina. "How to Connect with Your Higher Self, According to Mindvalley's Spirituality Teachers." Mindvalley, May 10, 2022. https://blog.mindvalley.com/higher-self/#h-what-is-your-higher-self.

Chapter 3—Your Body Remembers Your Trauma

American Psychological Association. "Stress Effects on the Body." March 8, 2023. https://www.apa.org/topics/stress/body.

Barker, D. J. "The Fetal and Infant Origins of Adult Disease." *British Medical Journal/ British Medical Association* 301 (1990): 1111.

Boccia, Maddalena, Laura Piccardi, and Paola Guariglia. "The Meditative Mind: A Comprehensive Meta-Analysis of MRI Studies." *Biomedical Research International* (2015): 11.

Bonaz, Bruno, Valérie Sinniger, and Sonia Pellissier. "Anti-Inflammatory Properties of the Vagus Nerve: Potential Therapeutic Implications of Vagus Nerve Stimulation." *Journal of Physiology* 594, no. 20 (2016): 5781–5790.

———. "The Vagus Nerve in the Neuro-Immune Axis: Implications in the Pathology of the Gastrointestinal Tract." *Frontiers in Immunology* 8 (2017): 1452.

Bourzat, Françoise, and Kristina Hunter. *Consciousness Medicine: Indigenous Wisdom, Entheogens, and Expanded States of Consciousness for Healing and Growth.* Berkeley: North Atlantic Books, 2019.

Bullmore, Edward. *The Inflamed Mind: A Radical New Approach to Depression.* New York: Picador, 2018.

Campbell, Jennifer A., Rebekah J. Walker, and Leonard E. Egede. "Associations between Adverse Childhood Experiences, High-Risk Behaviors, and Morbidity in Adulthood." *American Journal of Preventive Medicine* 50, no. 3 (2016): 344–352.

Center on the Developing Child at Harvard University. *InBrief: Connecting the Brain to the Rest of the Body.* 2021. https://developingchild.harvard.edu/resources/inbrief -connecting-the-brain-to-the-rest-of-the-body/.

Collins, Stephen M. "Stress and the Gastrointestinal Tract IV. Modulation of Intestinal Inflammation by Stress: Basic Mechanisms and Clinical Relevance." *American Journal of Physiology: Gastrointestinal and Liver Physiology* 280, no. 3 (2001): G315–G318.

Hays, Seth A., Robert L. Rennaker, and Michael P. Kilgard. "Targeting Plasticity with Vagus Nerve Stimulation to Treat Neurological Disease." *Progress in Brain Research* 207 (2013): 275–299.

Jones, Heather. "Understanding the Body's Stress Response." *Verywell Health*, June 21, 2022. https://www.verywellhealth.com/stress-hormones-5224662.

Jungmann, Manuela, Shervin Vencatachellum, Dimitri Van Ryckeghem, and Claus Vögele. "Effects of Cold Stimulation on Cardiac-Vagal Activation in Healthy Participants: Randomized Controlled Trial." *Journal of Medical Internet Research* 2, no. 2 (2018): e10257.

Kelly, John R., Paul J. Kennedy, John F. Cryan, Timothy G. Dinan, Gerard Clarke, and Niall P. Hyland. "Breaking Down the Barriers: The Gut Microbiome, Intestinal Permeability and Stress-Related Psychiatric Disorders." *Frontiers in Cellular Neuroscience* 9 (2015): 392.

Kempuraj, Duraisamy, Ramasamy Thangavel, Prashant A. Natteru, Govindhasamy P. Selvakumar, Daniyal Saeed, H. Zahoor, Smita Zaheer, S. Shankar Iyer, and Asgar Zaheer. "Neuroinflammation Induces Neurodegeneration." *Journal of Neurology, Neurosurgery and Spine* 1, no. 1 (2016): 1003.

Kendall-Tackett, Kathleen. *The Psychoneuroimmunology of Chronic Disease: Exploring the Links between Inflammation, Stress, and Illness.* Washington, DC: American Psychological Association, 2009.

Korb, Alex. *The Upward Spiral: Using Neuroscience to Reverse the Course of Depression, One Small Change at a Time.* Oakland: New Harbinger Publications, 2015.

Lupien, Sonia J., Charles W. Wilkinson, Sophie Brière, Catherine Ménard, Ng Mien Kwong Ng Kin, and Nayana Nair. "The Modulatory Effects of Corticosteroids on Cognition: Studies in Young Human Populations." *Psychoneuroendocrinology* 27 (2002): 401–416.

Macgill, Markus. "Alzheimer's Disease: Symptoms, Stages, Causes, and Treatments." *Medical News Today,* September 3, 2020. https://www.medicalnewstoday.com /articles/159442.

Maté, Gabor. *When the Body Says No: The Cost of Hidden Stress.* Pontiac: Scribe, 2003.

Nabavizadeh, Fatemeh, Mohammad Vahedian, Hedayat Sahraei, Soheila Adeli, and Ehsan Salimi. "Physical and Psychological Stress Have Similar Effects on Gastric Acid and Pepsin Secretions in Rat." *Journal of Stress Physiological Biochemistry* 7 (2011): 164–174.

Nakazawa, Donna J. *Childhood Disrupted: How Your Biography Becomes Your Biology, and How You Can Heal.* New York: Atria Books, 2016.

Naveen, Gupta H., Shivarama Varambally, Jagadisha Thirthalli, Mukund Rao, Rita Christopher, and B. N. Gangadhar. "Serum Cortisol and BDNF in Patients with Major Depression-Effect of Yoga." *International Review of Psychiatry* 28, no. 3 (2016): 273–278.

Nerurkar, Aditi, Asaf Bitton, Roger B. Davis, Russell S. Phillips, and Gloria Yeh. "When Physicians Counsel About Stress: Results of a National Study." *Journal of the American Medical Association—Internal Medicine* 173, no. 1 (2013): 76–77.

Nguyen, Kathy. "Echoic Survivals: Re-documenting Pre-1975 Vietnamese Music as Historical Sound/Tracks of Remembering." *Violence: An International Journal* 1, no. 2 (2020): 303–331.

Nicholson, Jeremy K., Elaine Holmes, and Ian D. Wilson. "Gut Microorganisms, Mammalian Metabolism and Personalized Health Care." *Nature Reviews—Microbiology* 3 (2005): 431–438.

Osanloo, Naser, Naheed Sarahian, Homeira Zardooz, Hedayat Sahraei, Mohammad Sahraei, and Bahareh Sadeghi. "Effects of Memantine, an NMDA Antagonist, on Metabolic Syndromes in Female NMRI Mice." *Basic and Clinical Neuroscience* 6, no. 4 (2015): 239–252.

Pembrey, Marcus. "A Whiff of Fear Down the Generations." Progress Education Trust, December 9, 2013. https://www.progress.org.uk/a-whiff-of-fear-down-the -generations/.

Pietrangelo, Ann. "The Effects of Stress on Your Body." Healthline, March 21, 2023. https://www.healthline.com/health/stress/effects-on-body#Central-nervous-and -endocrine-systems.

Qin, Hong-Yan, Chung-Wah Cheng, Xu-Dong Tang, and Zhao-Xiang Bian. "Impact of Psychological Stress on Irritable Bowel Syndrome." *World Journal of Gastroenterology* 20, no. 39 (2014): 14126–14131.

Ramsey, Drew. *Eat to Beat Depression and Anxiety: Nourish Your Way to Better Mental Health in Six Weeks.* New York: Harper Wave, 2021.

Sarahian, Nahid, Hedayat Sahraei, Homeira Zardooz, Hengamet Alibeik, and Baharet Sadeghi. "Effect of Memantine Administration within the Nucleus Accumbens on Changes in Weight and Volume of the Brain and Adrenal Gland During Chronic Stress in Female Mice." *Modares Journal of Medical Sciences: Pathobiology* 17 (2014): 71–82.

Segerstrom, Suzanne C., and Gregory E. Miller. "Psychological Stress and the Human Immune System: A Meta-analytic Study of 30 Years of Inquiry." *Psychology Bulletin* 130, no. 4 (2004): 601–630.

Shonkoff, Jack P. *Re-envisioning Early Childhood Policy and Practice in a World of Striking Inequality and Uncertainty.* Center on the Developing Child at Harvard University, January 2022. https://developingchild.harvard.edu/re-envisioning-ecd/.

Tabish, Syed, A. "Complementary and Alternative Healthcare: Is It Evidence-Based?" *International Journal of Health Sciences* 2, no. 1 (2008), v–ix.

van der Kolk, Bessel. *The Body Keeps the Score: Brain, Mind, and Body in the Healing of Trauma.* New York: Penguin Publishing Group, 2014.

Yaribeygi, Habib, Yunes Panahi, Hedayat Sahraei, Thomas, P. Johnston, and Amirhossein Sahebkar. "The Impact of Stress on Body Function: A Review." *Experimental and Clinical Sciences Journal* 16 (2017): 1057–1072.

Yuan, Haidan, Qianqian Ma, Li Ye, and Guangchun Piao. "The Traditional Medicine and Modern Medicine from Natural Products." *Molecules* 21, no. 5 (2016): 559.

Chapter 4—Unhealed Trauma and You

Bowers, Mallory, and Rachel Yehuda. "Intergenerational Transmission of Stress in Humans." *Neuropsychopharmacology* 41 (2016): 232–244.

Copping, Valerie. *Re-circuiting Trauma Pathways in Adults, Parents, and Children.* New York: Routledge, 2018.

Coyle, Sue. "Intergenerational Trauma—Legacies of Loss." *Social Work Today* 14 (2014): 18.

Cunningham, Ashley M., Deena M. Walker, Aarthi Ramakrishnan, Marie A. Doyle, Rosemary C. Bagot, Hannah M. Cates, Catherine J. Peña, Orna Issler, Casey K. Lardner, Caleb Browne, Scott J. Russo, Li Shen, and Eric J. Nestler. "Sperm Transcriptional State Associated with Paternal Transmission of Stress Phenotypes." *Journal of Neuroscience* 41 (2021): 6202–6216.

Franco, Fabiana. "Understanding Intergenerational Trauma: An Introduction for Clinicians." *GoodTherapy*, January 8, 2021. https://www.goodtherapy.org/blog/Understanding_Intergenerational_Trauma.

Herman, Judith L. *Trauma and Recovery.* New York: Basic Books, 1997.

Houck, James A. *When Ancestors Weep: Healing the Soul from Intergenerational Trauma.* Bloomington: Abbott Press, 2018.

Isobel, Sophie, Melinda Goodyear, Trentham Furness, and Kim Foster. "Preventing Intergenerational Trauma Transmission: A Critical Interpretive Synthesis." *Journal of Clinical Nursing* 28, nos. 7–8 (2019): 1100–1113.

Leal, Melissa, Beth R. Middleton and M. Moreno. *Intergenerational Trauma and Healing.* Basel: MDPI, 2021.

Lipton, Bruce H. *The Biology of Belief: Unleashing the Power of Consciousness, Matter & Miracles.* Carlsbad, CA: Hay House, 2016.

Lumey, Lambert H., Aryeh D. Stein, Henry S. Kahn, Karin M. van der Pal-de Bruin, Gerard J. Blauw, Patricia A. Zybert, and Ezra S. Susser. "The Dutch Hunger Winter." *International Journal of Epidemiology* 36, no. 6 (2007): 1196–1204.

Maracle, Lee. *First Wives Club: Coast Salish Style.* Penticton, BC: Theytus Books, 2010.

Perroud, Nader P., Eugene Rutembesa, Ariane Paoloni-Giacobino, Jean Mutabaruka, Léon Mutesa, Ludwig Stenz, Alain Malafosse, and Félicien Karege. "The Tutsi Genocide and Transgenerational Transmission of Maternal Stress: Epigenetics and Biology of the HPA Axis." *World Journal of Biological Psychiatry* 15, no. 4 (2014): 334–345.

Perry, Bruce, and Oprah Winfrey. *What Happened to You? Conversations on Trauma, Resilience, and Healing.* New York: Flatiron Books, 2021.

Somé, Malidoma P. *The Healing Wisdom of Africa: Finding Life Purpose Through Nature, Ritual, and Community.* New York: TarcherPerigee, 1999.

Waretini-Karena, Rāwiri. "Transforming Māori Experiences of Historical Intergenerational Trauma." PhD thesis, Te Whare Wānanga o Awanuiārangi Indigenous University, 2014.

Wolynn, Mark. *It Didn't Start with You: How Inherited Family Trauma Shapes Who We Are and How to End the Cycle.* New York: Penguin Publishing Group, 2017.

Yehuda, Rachel, Sarah L. Halligan, and Robert Grossman. "Childhood Trauma and Risk for PTSD: Relationship to Intergenerational Effects of Trauma, Parental PTSD, and Cortisol Excretion." *Development and Psychopathology* 13, no. 3 (2001): 733–753.

Yehuda, Rachel, Stephanie Mulherin Engel, Sarah R. Brand, Jonathan Seckl, Sue M. Marcus, and Gertrude S. Berkowitz. "Transgenerational Effects of Posttraumatic Stress Disorder in Babies of Mothers Exposed to the World Trade Center Attacks During Pregnancy." *Journal of Clinical Endocrinology & Metabolism* 90, no. 7 (2005): 4115–4118.

Yehuda, Rachel, and Amy Lehrner. "Intergenerational Transmission of Trauma Effects: Putative Role of Epigenetic Mechanisms." *World Psychiatry* 17, no. 3 (2018): 243–257.

Chapter 5—A Genetic Inheritance

Barker, David J. P. *Mothers, Babies and Health in Later Life.* London: Churchill Livingstone, 1998.

Bernard-Bonnin, Anne-Claude. "Maternal Depression and Child Development." *Paediatrics & Child Health* 9, no. 8 (2004): 575–583.

Conradt, Elisabeth, Daniel E. Adkins, Sheila Crowell, Catherine Monk, and Michael S. Kobor. "An Epigenetic Pathway Approach to Investigating Associations between Prenatal Exposure to Maternal Mood Disorder and Newborn Neurobehavior." *Developmental Psychopathology* 30, no. 3 (2018): 881–890.

Cummings, E. Mark, and Patrick T. Davies. "Maternal Depression and Child Development." *Journal of Child Psychology and Psychiatry* 35, no. 1 (1994): 73–112.

Cunningham, Ashley M., Deena M. Walker, Aarthi Ramakrishnan, Marie A. Doyle, Rosemary C. Bagot, Hannah M. Cates, Catherine J. Peña, Orna Issler, Casey K. Lardner, Caleb Browne, Scott J. Russo, Li Shen, and Eric J. Nestler. "Sperm Transcriptional State Associated with Paternal Transmission of Stress Phenotypes." *Journal of Neuroscience* 41 (2021): 6202–6216.

Dispenza, Joe. *Breaking the Habit of Being Yourself: How to Lose Your Mind and Create a New One.* Carlsbad: Hay House, 2013.

Franklin, Tamara B., Holger Russig, Isabelle C. Weiss, Johannes Graff, Natcha Linder, Aubin Michalon, Sandor Vizi, and Isabelle M. Mansuy. "Epigenetic Transmission of the Impact of Early Stress across Generations." *Biological Psychiatry* 68 (2010): 408–415.

Gapp, Katharina, Ali Jawaid, Peter Sarkies, Johannes Bohacek, Pawel Pelczar, Juliene Prados, Laurent Farinelli, Eric Miska, and Isabelle M. Mansuy. "Implication of Sperm RNAs in Transgenerational Inheritance of the Effects of Early Trauma in Mice." *Nature Neuroscience* 17 (2014): 667–669.

Gustafson, Craig. "Bruce Lipton, PhD: The Jump from Cell Culture to Consciousness." *Integrative Medicine* 16, no. 6 (2017): 44–50.

Houck, Patrick A. *When Ancestors Weep: Healing the Soul from Intergenerational Trauma.* Austin: Abbott Press, 2018.

Hui, Alyssa. "How Does Stress Impact Different Parts of the Body?" *Verywell Health,* April 5, 2023. https://www.verywellhealth.com/how-does-stress-affect-different-parts-of-the-body-7375233.

Levine, Peter A. *Waking the Tiger: Healing Trauma.* Berkeley: North Atlantic Books, 1997.

Liang Yiming, Zhao Yiming, Zhou Yueyue, and Liu Zhengkui. "How Maternal Trauma Exposure Contributed to Children's Depressive Symptoms following the Wenchuan Earthquake: A Multiple Mediation Model Study." *International Journal of Environmental Research Public Health* 19, no. 24 (2022): 16881.

Lismer, Ariane, Vanessa Dumeaux, Christine Lafleur, Romain Lambrot, Julie Brind'Amour, Matthew C. Lorincz, and Sarah Kimmins. "Histone H3 Lysine 4 Trimethylation in Sperm Is Transmitted to the Embryo and Associated with Diet-Induced Phenotypes in the Offspring." *Developmental Cell* 56, no. 5 (2021): 671–686.

Lupien, Sonia J., Charles W. Wilkinson, Sophie Brière, Catherine Ménard, Ng Y. Kin, and Nibu P. Nair. "The Modulatory Effects of Corticosteroids on Cognition: Studies in Young Human Populations." *Psychoneuroendocrinology* 27 (2002): 401–416.

MacBride, Katie. "Can You Inherit Stress? Sperm Study Reveals Link to Mood." *Inverse,* June 7, 2021. https://www.inverse.com/mind-body/generational-mood-disorders-study.

Marsh, Jason. "Do Mirror Neurons Give Us Empathy?" *Greater Good Magazine,* March 29, 2012. https://greatergood.berkeley.edu/article/item/do_mirror_neurons_give_empathy.

Maté, Gabor. *When the Body Says No: The Cost of Hidden Stress.* Austin: Scribe, 2003.

National Scientific Council on the Developing Child. "Early Experiences Can Alter Gene Expression and Affect Long-Term Development." 2010. https://harvardcenter.wpenginepowered.com/wp-content/uploads/2010/05/Early-Experiences-Can-Alter-Gene-Expression-and-Affect-Long-Term-Development.pdf.

Švorcová, Jana. "Transgenerational Epigenetic Inheritance of Traumatic Experience in Mammals." *Genes* 14, no. 1 (2023):120.

Thumfart, Kristina M., Ali Jawaid, Kristina Bright, Marc Flachsmann, and Isabelle M. Mansuy. "Epigenetics of Childhood Trauma: Long Term Sequelae and Potential for Treatment." *Neuroscience and Biobehavioral Reviews* 132 (2022): 1049–1066.

van der Kolk, Bessel. *The Body Keeps the Score: Brain, Mind, and Body in the Healing of Trauma.* New York: Penguin Publishing Group, 2014.

Van Steenwyk, Gretchen, and Isabelle M. Mansuy. "Epigenetics and the Impact of Early-Life Stress across Generations." *Stress: Genetics, Epigenetics and Genomics* 4 (2021): 297–307.

Wolynn, Mark. *It Didn't Start with You: How Inherited Family Trauma Shapes Who We Are and How to End the Cycle.* New York: Penguin Publishing Group, 2017.

Yehuda, Rachel, and Linda M. Bierer. "The Relevance of Epigenetics to PTSD: Implications for the DSM-V." *Journal of Trauma Stress* 22 (2009): 427–434.

Yehuda, Rachel, Stephanie Mulherin Engel, Sarah R. Brand, Jonathan Seckl, Sue M. Marcus, and Gertrude S. Berkowitz. "Transgenerational Effects of Posttraumatic Stress Disorder in Babies of Mothers Exposed to the World Trade Center Attacks During Pregnancy." *Journal of Clinical Endocrinology & Metabolism* 90, no. 7 (2005): 4115–4118.

Yehuda, Rachel, and Amy Lehrner. "Intergenerational Transmission of Trauma Effects: Putative Role of Epigenetic Mechanisms." *World Psychiatry* 17, no. 3 (2018): 243–257.

Chapter 6—Your Intergenerational Nervous System

Baack, Gita A. *The Inheritors: Moving Forward from Generational Trauma.* Berkeley: She Writes Press, 2017.

Center on the Developing Child at Harvard University. *InBrief: Connecting the Brain to the Rest of the Body.* 2021. https://developingchild.harvard.edu/resources/inbrief -connecting-the-brain-to-the-rest-of-the-body/.

Dias, Brian G., and Kerri J. Ressler. "Parental Olfactory Experience Influences Behavior and Neural Structure in Subsequent Generations." *Nature Neuroscience* 17 (2014): 89–96.

Ghai, Meenu, and Farzeen Kader. "A Review on Epigenetic Inheritance of Experiences in Humans." *Biochemical Genetics* 60 (2022): 1107–1140.

Gray, Richard. "Phobias May Be Memories Passed Down in Genes from Ancestors." *Telegraph*, December 1, 2013. https://www.telegraph.co.uk/news/science/science -news/10486479/Phobias-may-be-memories-passed-down-in-genes-from -ancestors.html.

Greeson, Katherine W., Krista M. S. Crow, Clayton Edenfield, and Charles A. Easley IV. "Inheritance of Paternal Lifestyles and Exposures through Sperm DNA Methylation." *Nature Reviews Urology* 20, no. 6 (2023): 356–370.

Houck, Patrick A. *When Ancestors Weep: Healing the Soul from Intergenerational Trauma.* Austin: Abbott Press, 2018.

Nam, Min-Ho, Kwang S. Ahn, and Seung-Hoon Choi. "Acupuncture Stimulation Induces Neurogenesis in Adult Brain." *International Review of Neurobiology* 111 (2013): 67–90.

National Scientific Council on the Developing Child. "Early Experiences Can Alter Gene Expression and Affect Long-Term Development." 2010. https://harvardcenter .wpenginepowered.com/wp-content/uploads/2010/05/Early-Experiences-Can -Alter-Gene-Expression-and-Affect-Long-Term-Development.pdf.

Pembrey, Marcus. "A Whiff of Fear down the Generations." Progress Education Trust, December 9, 2013. https://www.progress.org.uk/a-whiff-of-fear-down-the -generations/.

Raccanello, Daniella, Camilla Gobbo, Lavinia Corona, Giorgia De Bona, Rob Hall, and Robert Burro. "Long-Term Intergenerational Transmission of Memories of the Vajont Disaster." *Psychological Trauma: Theory, Research, Practice, and Policy* 14, no. 7 (2022): 1107–1116.

Serpeloni, Fernanda, Karl Radtke, Simone G. de Assis, Federico Henning, Daniel Nätt, and Thomas Elbert. "Grandmaternal Stress During Pregnancy and DNA Methylation of the Third Generation: An Epigenome-Wide Association Study." *Translational Psychiatry* 7 (2017): 1202.

Shonkoff, Jack P. *Re-envisioning Early Childhood Policy and Practice in a World of Striking Inequality and Uncertainty.* Center on the Developing Child at Harvard University, January 2022. https://developingchild.harvard.edu/re-envisioning-ecd/.

Siegel, Daniel J. *The Developing Mind: How Relationships and the Brain Interact to Shape Who We Are.* New York: Guilford Press, 2012.

University of Haifa. "Unspoken Memories of Holocaust Survivors Find Silent and Nonpathological Expression." *ScienceDaily*, June 22, 2009. https://www.sciencedaily .com/releases/2009/06/090622103823.htm.

Walsh, Colleen. "What the Nose Knows." *Harvard Gazette*, February 27, 2020. https://news.harvard.edu/gazette/story/2020/02/how-scent-emotion-and-memory-are-intertwined-and-exploited/.

Wellness McUniverse. "EFT Tapping Points and Recipe." 2020. https://wellness.mcuniverse.com/eft-tapping-points-recipe/.

Yehuda, Rachel, Stephanie M. Engel, Sarah R. Brand, Jonathan Seckl, Sue M. Marcus, and Gertrud S. Berkowitz. "Transgenerational Effects of Posttraumatic Stress Disorder in Babies of Mothers Exposed to the World Trade Center Attacks During Pregnancy." *Journal of Clinical Endocrinology & Metabolism* 90, no. 7 (2005): 4115–4118.

Chapter 7—Your Intergenerational Inner Child

Ainsworth, Mary D. S., Mary C. Blehar, Everett Waters, and Sally Wall. *Patterns of Attachment: A Psychological Study of the Strange Situation*. Mahwah: Erlbaum, 1978.

Archer, Caroline. *Reparenting the Child Who Hurts: A Guide to Healing Developmental Trauma and Attachments*. Philadelphia: Jessica Kingsley Publishers, 2013.

Baron-Cohen, Simon, Michael Lombardo, and Helen Tager-Flusberg. *Understanding Other Minds: Perspectives from Developmental Social Neuroscience*. New York: Oxford University Press, 2013.

Bernard-Bonnin, Anne-Claude. "Maternal Depression and Child Development." *Paediatrics & Child Health* 9, no. 8 (2004): 575–583.

Bowlby, John. *Attachment and Loss*, Vol. 1, *Attachment*. New York: Basic Books, 1969, 1982.

Burke Harris, Nadine. *The Deepest Well: Healing the Long-Term Effects of Childhood Trauma and Adversity*. New York: Mariner Books, 2018.

Campbell, Jennifer A., Rebekah J. Walker, and Leonard E. Egede. "Associations between Adverse Childhood Experiences, High-Risk Behaviors, and Morbidity in Adulthood." *American Journal of Preventive Medicine* 50, no. 3 (2016): 344–352.

Chang Ha, Betsy. *The Paper Tiger's Daughters: A Self-Healing Journey to Stop the Generational and Intersectional Harm of ACEs in the AAPI Community*. Self-published, 2022.

Cicchetti, Dante, Fred A. Rogosch, and Sheree L. Toth. "Fostering Secure Attachment in Infants in Maltreating Families through Preventive Interventions." *Development and Psychopathology* 18, no. 3 (2006): 623–649.

Cummings, E. Mark, and Patrick T. Davies. "Maternal Depression and Child Development." *Journal of Child Psychology and Psychiatry* 35, no. 1 (1994): 73–112.

Escueta, Maya. "The Economics and Child Development Science of Intergenerational Trauma." Columbia Academic Commons, 2021. https://academiccommons.columbia.edu/doi/10.7916/d8-a8xg-fk13.

Forward, Susan, with C. F. Buck. *Toxic Parents: Overcoming Their Hurtful Legacy and Reclaiming Your Life*. New York: Bantam Books, 1989.

Gibson, Lindsay C. *Adult Children of Emotionally Immature Parents: How to Heal from Distant, Rejecting, or Self-Involved Parents*. Oakland: New Harbinger Publications, 2015.

Graham, Linda. "The Power of Mindful Empathy to Heal Toxic Shame." 2020. https://lindagraham-mft.net/pdf/WiseBrainBulletin-4-1.pdf.

Hardie-Williams, Kathy. "Emotional Incest: When Parents Make Their Kids Partners." *GoodTherapy*, September 15, 2016. https:// www.goodtherapy.org/blog/emotional-covert-incest-when-parents-make- their-kids-partners-0914165.

Heller, Laurence, and Aline LaPierre. *Healing Developmental Trauma: How Early Trauma Affects Self-Regulation, Self-Image, and the Capacity for Relationship.* Berkeley: North Atlantic Books, 2012.

Hosseini, Khaled. *The Kite Runner.* New York: Riverhead Books, 2003.

Houck, James A. *When Ancestors Weep: Healing the Soul from Intergenerational Trauma.* Bloomington: Abbott Press, 2018.

Lyons-Ruth, Karlen. "Dissociation and the Parent–Infant Dialogue: A Longitudinal Perspective from Attachment Research." *Journal of the American Psychoanalytic Association* 51, no. 3 (2003): 883–911.

Nakazawa, Donna J. *Childhood Disrupted: How Your Biography Becomes Your Biology, and How You Can Heal.* New York: Atria Books, 2016.

Perry, Philippa. *The Book You Wish Your Parents Had Read: And Your Children Will Be Glad That You Did.* New York: Penguin Life, 2020.

Porges, Stephen. *The Pocket Guide to Polyvagal Theory.* New York: W. W. Norton & Company, 2017.

Sack, David. "When Emotional Trauma Is a Family Affair." *Psychology Today*, May 5, 2014. https://www.psychologytoday.com/us/blog/where-science-meets-the-steps/201405/when-emotional-trauma-is-family-affair.

Siegel, Daniel J. *The Developing Mind: How Relationships and the Brain Interact to Shape Who We Are.* New York: Guilford Press, 2012.

Simonelli, Alessandra, and Micol Parolin. "Strange Situation Test." In *Encyclopedia of Personality and Individual Differences*, edited by Virgil Zeigler-Hill and Todd Shackelford. New York: Springer, 2016.

Wang, X. "Breaking the Cycle of Intergenerational Trauma." PhD diss., Ohio State University, 2019.

Williams, Lewis. *Indigenous Intergenerational Resilience: Confronting Cultural and Ecological Crisis.* New York: Routledge, 2022.

Chapter 8—Intergenerational Cycles of Abuse

Alexander, Pamela C. *Intergenerational Cycles of Trauma and Violence: An Attachment and Family Systems Perspective.* New York: W. W. Norton & Company, 2014.

Beattie, Melody. *Codependent No More: How to Stop Controlling Others and Start Caring for Yourself.* Center City: Hazelden, 1987.

Burke Harris, Nadine. *The Deepest Well: Healing the Long-Term Effects of Childhood Trauma and Adversity.* New York: Mariner Books, 2018.

Edleson, Jeffrey. "Cycle of Violence." In *Encyclopedia of Interpersonal Violence*, Vol. 1, edited by Claire M. Renzetti and Jeffrey L. Edleson, 166. Thousand Oaks, CA: SAGE Publications, 2008.

Francis, Elizabeth M. "Eating a Can of Worms: Treating Transgenerational Trauma in Middle Eastern Women." PhD diss., Pacifica Graduate Institute, 2022.

Forward, Susan, with Craig F. Buck. *Toxic Parents: Overcoming Their Hurtful Legacy and Reclaiming Your Life.* New York: Bantam Books, 1989.

Graham, Linda. "The Power of Mindful Empathy to Heal Toxic Shame." 2020. https://lindagraham-mft.net/pdf/WiseBrainBulletin-4-1.pdf.

hooks, bell. *All about Love: New Visions.* New York: William Morrow, 2000.

King, R. *Healing Rage: Women Making Inner Peace Possible.* New York: Avery, 2008.

Lyon, Bret. "Shame and Trauma." Center for Healing Shame, August 21, 2017. https://healingshame.com/articles/2017/8/21/shame-and-trauma.

MacKenzie, J. *Psychopath Free: Recovering from Emotionally Abusive Relationships with Narcissists, Sociopaths, and Other Toxic People.* New York: Berkley Books, 2015.

Matsakis, Aphrodite. *Loving Someone with PTSD: A Practical Guide to Understanding and Connecting with Your Partner after Trauma.* Oakland: New Harbinger Publications, 2013.

Moylan, Carrie A., Todd I. Herrenkohl, Cindy Sousa, Emiko A. Tajima, Roy C. Herrenkohl, and Jean M. Russo. "The Effects of Child Abuse and Exposure to Domestic Violence on Adolescent Internalizing and Externalizing Behavior Problems." *Journal of Family Violence* 25, no. 1 (2010): 53–63.

Snarr, Jeffrey, Amy Smith Slep, and Richard Heyman. "Intergenerational Transmission of Abuse." In *Encyclopedia of Human Relationships*, edited by Harry T. Reis and Susan Sprecher, 876–878. Thousand Oaks: SAGE Publications, 2009.

Chapter 9—When Collective Trauma Enters Your Home

Abramson, Ashley. "Substance Use During the Pandemic." American Psychological Association, March 1, 2021. https://www.apa.org/monitor/2021/03/substance-use-pandemic.

Agyapong, Belinda, Reham Shalaby, Ejamai Eboreime, Gloria Obuobi-Donkor, Ernest Owusu, Menard K. Adu, Wanying Mao, Folajinmi Oluwasina, and Vincent I. O. Agyaponga. "Cumulative Trauma from Multiple Natural Disasters Increases Mental Health Burden on Residents of Fort McMurray." *European Journal of Psychotraumatology* 13, no. 1 (2022): 2059999.

Barker, Joanne. "Racism Is a Health Issue: How It Affects Kids, What Parents Can Do." Boston Children's Hospital, June 10, 2020. https://answers.childrenshospital.org/racism-child-health/.

Caruso, Germán D. "The Legacy of Natural Disasters: The Intergenerational Impact of 100 Years of Disasters in Latin America." *Journal of Development Economics* 127(C) (2017): 209–233.

Cohen, Sandy. "Oprah Winfrey, U.S. Surgeon General Vivek Murthy headline WOW 2023 Mental Health Summit." *UCLA Health*, May 4, 2023. https://www.uclahealth.org/news/oprah-winfrey-us-surgeon-general-vivek-murthy-headline-wow#:~:text="Mental%20health%20is%20the%20defining,4%20at%20UCLA%27s%20Royce%20Hall.

Columb, David, Raza Hussain, and Colin O'Gara. "Addiction Psychiatry and COVID-19: Impact on Patients and Service Provision." *Irish Journal of Psychological Medicine* 37, no. 3 (2020): 164–168.

Czeisler, Mark É., Rashon I. Lane, Emiko Petrosky, et al. "Mental Health, Substance Use, and Suicidal Ideation During the COVID-19 Pandemic—United States." *Morbidity and Mortality Weekly Report* 69, Centers for Disease Control (2020): 1049–1057.

DeGruy Leary, Joy. *Post Traumatic Slave Syndrome: America's Legacy of Enduring Injury and Healing.* Baltimore: Uptone Press, 2005.

Deoni, Sean C., Jennifer Beauchemin, Alexandra Volpe, and Viren Dâ Sa. "Impact of the COVID-19 Pandemic on Early Child Cognitive Development: Initial Findings in a Longitudinal Observational Study of Child Health." *MedRxiv* 5 (2021): 13.

Der Sarkissian, Alissa, and Jill D. Sharkey. "Transgenerational Trauma and Mental Health Needs among Armenian Genocide Descendants." *International Journal of Environmental Research and Public Health* 18, no. 19 (2021): 10554.

DeWolf, Thomas N., and Jodie Geddes. *The Little Book of Racial Healing: Coming to the Table for Truth-Telling, Liberation, and Transformation.* Newark: Good Books, 2019.

Dyer, Owen "Covid-19: Children Born During the Pandemic Score Lower on Cognitive Tests, Study Finds." *British Medical Journal/British Medical Association* 374 (2021): n2031.

Ellis, Wendy R., and William H. Dietz. "A New Framework for Addressing Adverse Childhood and Community Experiences: The Building Community Resilience Model." *Academic Pediatrics* 17, no. 7S (2017): S86–S93.

Gindt, Morgane, Arnaud Fernandez, Aurelien Richez, Ophelie Nachon, Michele Battista, and Florence Askenazy. "CoCo20 Protocol: A Pilot Longitudinal Follow-Up Study about the Psychiatric Outcomes in a Paediatric Population and Their Families During and after the Stay-at-Home Related to Coronavirus Pandemic (COVID-19)." *BMJ Open* 11, no. 4 (2021): e044667.

Goodnough, Abby. "Overdose Deaths Have Surged During the Pandemic, C.D.C. Data Shows." *New York Times*, April 4, 2021. https://www.nytimes.com/2021/04/14/health/overdose-deaths-fentanyl-opiods-coronaviurs-pandemic.html.

Haines, Staci K. *The Politics of Trauma.* Berkeley: North Atlantic Books, 2019.

Hesman, Judy, Marinus H. Van Ijzendoorn, and Abraham Sagi-Schwartz. "Cross-Cultural Patterns of Attachment: Universal and Contextual Dimensions." In *Handbook of Attachment: Theory, Research, and Clinical Applications*, edited by J. Cassidy and P. R. Shaver, 880–905. New York: Guilford Press, 2008.

Hirschberger, Gilad. "Collective Trauma and the Social Construction of Meaning." *Frontiers in Psychology* 9 (2018): 1441.

Institute for Collective Trauma and Growth. "Phases of Disaster Response." 2023. https://www.ictg.org/phases-of-disaster-response.html.

Kidron, Carol A. "Embracing the Lived Memory of Genocide: Holocaust Survivor and Descendant Renegade Memory Work at the House of Being." *American Ethnologist* 37, no. 3 (2010): 429–451.

Magee, Rhonda V. *The Inner Work of Racial Justice: Healing Ourselves and Transforming Our Communities through Mindfulness.* New York: TarcherPerigee, 2019.

Mason, Rhapsody. "The Impact of Racism on Pediatric Mental Health." Illinois DocAssist, April 21, 2021. https://docassistillinois.org/2021/04/21/the-impact-of-racism-on-pediatric-mental-health/.

Menakem, Resmaa. *My Grandmother's Hands.* Las Vegas: Central Recovery Press, 2017.

Menzies, Karen. "Understanding the Australian Aboriginal Experience of Collective, Historical and Intergenerational Trauma." *International Social Work* 62, no. 6 (2019): 1522–1534.

Morin, Amy. "Is Spanking Children an Effective Consequence?" *Verywell Family*, September 20, 2022. https://www.verywellfamily.com/is-spanking-children-a-good-way-to-discipline-1094756.

Morsey, Leila, and Richard Rothstein. "Toxic Stress and Children's Outcomes: African American Children Growing Up Poor Are at Greater Risk of Disrupted Physiological Functioning and Depressed Academic Achievement." Economic Policy Institute, May 1, 2019. https://www.epi.org/publication/toxic-stress-and-childrens-outcomes-african-american-children-growing-up-poor-are-at-greater-risk-of-disrupted-physiological-functioning-and-depressed-academic-achievement/.

Pumariega, Andres J., Jo Youngsuhk, Brent Beck, and Mariam Rahmani. "Trauma and US Minority Children and Youth." *Current Psychiatry Reports* 24, no. 4 (2022): 285–295.

Rashkin, Esther. "The Haunted Child: Social Catastrophe, Phantom Transmissions, and the Aftermath of Collective Trauma." *Psychoanalytic Review* 86, no. 3 (1999): 433–453.

Richtel, Matt. "The Surgeon General's New Mission: Adolescent Mental Health." *New York Times*, March 21, 2023. https://www.nytimes.com/2023/03/21/health /surgeon-general-adolescents-mental-health.html.

Rupcich, Claudia, Irinia Gonzalez, and Karell Roxas. "Why Millennial Latinx Parents Are Saying Goodbye to Chancla Culture." *The Skimm*, September 23, 2022. https://www.theskimm.com/parenting/millennial-latinx-parenting.

Saad, Layla F. *Me and White Supremacy: Combat Racism, Change the World, and Become a Good Ancestor.* New York: Sourcebooks, 2020.

Sack, David. "When Emotional Trauma Is a Family Affair." *Psychology Today*, May 5, 2014. https://www.psychologytoday.com/us/blog/where-science-meets-the -steps/201405/when-emotional-trauma-is-family-affair.

Sangalang, Cindy C., and Cindy Vang. "Intergenerational Trauma in Refugee Families: A Systematic Review." *Journal of Immigrant Minority Health* 19, no. 3 (2017): 745–754.

Saul, Jack. *Collective Trauma, Collective Healing: Promoting Community Resilience in the Aftermath of Disaster.* New York: Routledge, 2022.

Shah, Pooja. "How Intergenerational Trauma Impacts the South Asian Community." *Teen Vogue*, August 30, 2022. https://www.teenvogue.com/story/how-intergenerational -trauma-impacts-the-south-asian-community.

Singh, Shweta, Deblina Roy, Krittika Sinha, Sheeba Parveen, Ginni Sharma, and Gunjan Joshi. "Impact of COVID-19 and Lockdown on Mental Health of Children and Adolescents: A Narrative Review with Recommendations." *Psychiatry Research* 293 (2020): 113429.

Skloot, Rebecca. *The Immortal Life of Henrietta Lacks.* New York: Crown, 2010.

Substance Abuse and Mental Health Services Administration. *Crisis Counseling Assistance and Training Program Guidance.* 2016. https://www.samhsa.gov/sites /default/files/images/fema-ccp-guidance.pdf.

Ungar, Michael. "Systemic Resilience: Principles and Processes for a Science of Change in Contexts of Adversity." *Ecology and Society* 23, no. 4 (2018): 34.

Vidal, Juan. "'La Chancla': Flip Flops as a Tool of Discipline." *Code Switch*, NPR, November 4, 2014. https://www.npr.org/sections/codeswitch/2014/11/04/361205792 /la-chancla-flip-flops-as-a-tool-of-discipline.

Washington, Harriet A. *Medical Apartheid: The Dark History of Medical Experimentation on Black Americans from Colonial Times to the Present.* New York: Anchor, 2006.

Winters, Mary-Frances. *Black Fatigue: How Racism Erodes the Mind, Body, and Spirit.* Oakland: Berrett-Koehler Publishers, 2020.

World Health Organization. "COVID-19 Pandemic Triggers 25% Increase in Prevalence of Anxiety and Depression Worldwide." March 2, 2022. https://www.who.int /news/item/02-03-2022-covid-19-pandemic-triggers-25-increase-in-prevalence -of-anxiety-and-depression-worldwide.

Zagorski, Nick. "COVID-19's Impact on Development Remains Unclear." *Psychiatric News*, March 28, 2022. https://psychnews.psychiatryonline.org/doi/10.1176 /appi.pn.2022.04.3.38.

Chapter 10—Grieving Your Traumatic Lineage

Foor, Daniel. *Ancestral Medicine: Rituals for Personal and Family Healing.* Rochester: Bear & Company, 2017.

Fruzzetti, Alan. *The High-Conflict Couple: A Dialectical Behavior Therapy Guide to Finding Peace, Intimacy, and Validation.* Oakland: New Harbinger Publications, 2006.

Graham, Linda. "The Power of Mindful Empathy to Heal Toxic Shame." 2020. https://lindagraham-mft.net/pdf/WiseBrainBulletin-4-1.pdf.

Mucci, Clara. *Beyond Individual and Collective Trauma: Intergenerational Transmission, Psychoanalytic Treatment, and the Dynamics of Forgiveness.* New York: Routledge, 2013.

Rankin, Lisa. *Sacred Medicine: A Doctor's Quest to Unravel the Mysteries of Healing.* Louisville: Sounds True, 2022.

Robertson, Patricia K. *Connect with Your Ancestors: Transforming the Transgenerational Trauma of Your Family Tree: Exploring Systemic Healing, Inherited Emotional Genealogy, Entanglements, Epigenetics and Body Focused Systemic Constellations.* Calgary: Peaceful Possibilities Press, 2018.

Winfrey, Oprah. *The Wisdom of Sundays: Life-Changing Insights from Super Soul Conversations.* New York: Macmillan, 2017.

Wolynn, Mark. *It Didn't Start with You: How Inherited Family Trauma Shapes Who We Are and How to End the Cycle.* New York: Penguin Publishing Group, 2017.

Yehuda, Rachel, and Amy Lehrner. "Intergenerational Transmission of Trauma Effects: Putative Role of Epigenetic Mechanisms." *World Psychiatry* 17, no. 3 (2018): 243–257.

Chapter 11—Embodying Generational Resilience

Houck, James A. *When Ancestors Weep: Healing the Soul from Intergenerational Trauma.* Bloomington: Abbott Press, 2018.

Kumai, Candice. *Kintsugi Wellness: The Japanese Art of Nourishing Mind, Body, and Spirit.* New York: Harper Wave, 2018.

Lamar, Kendrick. "DNA," *DAMN.* TDE; Aftermath; Interscope, 2017, compact disc.

Morin, Amy. *13 Things Mentally Strong People Don't Do: Take Back Your Power, Embrace Change, Face Your Fears, and Train Your Brain for Happiness and Success.* New York: William Morrow, 2017.

Nakazawa, Donna J. *Childhood Disrupted: How Your Biography Becomes Your Biology, and How You Can Heal.* New York: Atria Books, 2016.

Rankin, Lissa. *Sacred Medicine: A Doctor's Quest to Unravel the Mysteries of Healing.* Louisville: Sounds True, 2022.

Rowe, Sheila W., and Soong-Chan Rha. *Healing Racial Trauma: The Road to Resilience.* Westmont: IVP, 2020.

Schwartz, Arielle. *The Post-Traumatic Growth Guidebook: Practical Mind-Body Tools to Heal Trauma, Foster Resilience and Awaken Your Potential.* New York: Pesi Publishing Media, 2020.

Shevell, Meaghan C., and Myriam S. Denov. "A Multidimensional Model of Resilience: Family, Community, National, Global and Intergenerational Resilience." *Child Abuse & Neglect* 119, no. 2 (2021): 105035.

Tedeschi, Richard G., and Lawrence G. Calhoun. "The Posttraumatic Growth Inventory: Measuring the Positive Legacy of Trauma." *Journal of Traumatic Stress* 9, no. 3 (1996): 455–471.

Wolynn, Mark. *It Didn't Start with You: How Inherited Family Trauma Shapes Who We Are and How to End the Cycle.* New York: Penguin Publishing Group, 2017.

Chapter 12—Leaving a Generational Legacy

Cicchetti, Dante, Fred A. Rogosch, and Sheree L. Toth. "Fostering Secure Attachment in Infants in Maltreating Families through Preventive Interventions." *Development and Psychopathology* 18, no. 3 (2006): 623–649.

Coates, Susan W., Daniel S. Schechter, and Elsa First. "Brief Interventions with Traumatized Children and Families after September 11." In *September 11: Trauma and Human Bonds,* edited by Susan W. Coates, Jane L. Rosenthal, and Daniel S. Schechter, 23–49. New York: Analytic Press/Taylor & Francis Group, 2003.

Duncan, Alaine D., and Kathy L. Kain. *Tao of Trauma: A Practitioner's Guide for Integrating Five Element Theory and Trauma Treatment.* Berkeley: North Atlantic Books, 2019.

Gapp, Katharina, Johannes Bohacek, Jonas Grossmann, Andrea M. Brunner, Francesca Manuella, Paolo Nanni, and Isabelle M. Mansuy. "Potential of Environmental Enrichment to Prevent Transgenerational Effects of Paternal Trauma." *Neuropsychopharmacology* 41, no. 11 (2016): 2749–2758.

Grand, Sue. *The Hero in the Mirror: From Fear to Fortitude.* New York: Routledge, 2009.

Morgan, Patricia. "Intergenerational Resilience: Care*Communicate*Connect." Solutions for Resilience, n.d. https://www.solutionsforresilience.com/intergenerational -resilience/.

Schechter, Daniel S. "Intergenerational Communication of Maternal Violent Trauma: Understanding the Interplay of Reflective Functioning and Posttraumatic Psychopathology." In *September 11: Trauma and Human Bonds,* edited by Susan W. Coates, Jane L. Rosenthal, and Daniel S. Schechter, 115–142. New York: Routledge, 2013.

Schechter, Daniel S., Michael M. Myers, Susan A. Brunelli, Susan W. Coates, Charles H. Zeanah Jr., Mark Davies, John F. Grienenberger, Randall D. Marshall, Jaime E. McCaw, Kimberly A. Trabka, and Michael R. Liebowitz. "Traumatized Mothers Can Change Their Minds about Their Toddlers: Understanding How a Novel Use of Videofeedback Supports Positive Change of Maternal Attributions." *Infant Mental Health Journal* 27, no. 5 (2006): 429–447.

Schofield, Thomas J., Rand D. Conger, and Tricia K. Neppl. "Positive Parenting, Beliefs about Parental Efficacy, and Active Coping: Three Sources of Intergenerational Resilience." *Journal of Family Psychology* 28, no. 6 (2014): 973–978.

Shonkoff, Jack P. *Re-envisioning Early Childhood Policy and Practice in a World of Striking Inequality and Uncertainty.* Center on the Developing Child at Harvard University, January 2022. https://developingchild.harvard.edu/re-envisioning-ecd/.

Stein, Bradley D., Lisa H. Jaycox, Sheryl H. Kataoka, Marleen Wong, Wenli Tu, Marc N. Elliott, and Arlene Fink. "A Mental Health Intervention for Schoolchildren Exposed to Violence: A Randomized Controlled Trial." *JAMA: Journal of the American Medical Association* 290, no. 5 (2003): 603–611.

Williams, Lewis. *Indigenous Intergenerational Resilience: Confronting Cultural and Ecological Crisis.* New York: Routledge, 2022.

Index

Note: Italicized page numbers indicate material in tables or illustrations.

About the Author

Mariel Buqué, Ph.D., is a Columbia University–trained, trauma-informed psychologist, professor, and sound bath meditation healer. She received her doctorate in counseling psychology from Columbia University, where she also trained as a fellow in holistic mental health. Her clinical framework infuses ancient and Indigenous healing practices into a modern, comprehensive therapeutic approach. She has utilized her training in holistic care to integrate holistic practices, like sound bath meditation and breathwork, into therapy, which has helped to deepen trauma healing for an entire generation of clients. In addition, she provides healing workshops to Fortune 100 companies, including Google, Capital One, and Meta, and lectures within the psychology department at Columbia University. Dr. Buqué is widely sought out for her clinical expertise and trauma approach and has been featured on major media outlets, including *Today*, *Good Morning America*, and ABC News. She has been named as a School of Greatness's 100 Greatest People Doing Good and an inaugural Verywell Mind 25 Mental Health Champion. She is originally from the Dominican Republic and currently lives in New Jersey.

Her work can be found at drmarielbuque.com and @Dr.Mariel Buqué.